Congratulations!

YOU DON'T NEED A DIET, YOU NEED A HEALTH TRANSFORMATION FROM THE INSIDE OUT
- Dr. William Sears

RESTORE YOUR HEALTH. Enjoy a simple transition to clean eating and lifestyle habits that help you gain energy and strengthen your immune system. So, you can spend more time doing the things you love, with the people you love! Be the positive influence and role model that inspires your children or those around you to join this journey.

Achieve healthier and sustainable lifestyle habits by implementing simple steps each week outlined in this 52-week plan. Why 52 weeks? Because we're not looking for a 6 or 12-week challenge to get you started, we're looking to TRANSFORM YOUR LIVES for good. Through education and small weekly challenges carefully planned over one year, Nurse Coach Jade will help you and your family be on a road to living your healthiest life. Perfect for the busy family!

GREAT THINGS ARE DONE BY A SERIES OF
SMALL THINGS BROUGHT TOGETHER
- Vincent Van Gogh

You don't need tons of willpower to form new habits, but you do need patience, grace, and perseverance through the tough days. This is the ultimate definition of self-care as you learn to love yourself enough to truly understand your body's needs. The micro-decisions you make each day significantly impacts your future. Nurse Coach Jade will give you the tools to make these small changes each day, that will make a huge impact on your future health and well-being. Your future self will thank you!

GOOD LUCK ON YOUR JOURNEY!

Jade Padlan
Registered Nurse | Certified Health Coach

@anti.inflammatory.living   www.anti-inflammatoryliving.com   @antiinflammatoryliving

Join our Facebook group - Anti-Inflammatory Living Family - to meet others on the same journey!

EVERY TIME YOU
EAT OR DRINK
YOU ARE EITHER
Feeding Disease
OR
Fighting it

- Heather Morgan

just eat REAL foods

CLEAN EATING = HEALTHY FAMILY = HAPPY FAMILY

BE A POSITIVE INFLUENCE!

You will be confident your kids are investing in their future by teaching them the education and tips to incorporate healthier habits and behaviors in their life. This will serve your family for generations

NO MORE DIETS!

You will learn the unique nutrition requirements needed for your growing children to transform their health inside out. Learn to eat clean and combat inflammation & diseases. You will sleep better and FEEL GOOD

SHOP SMART

You will understand how to analyze nutrition food labels and ingredients list to purchase the cleanest foods that benefit your family's health, and not be fooled by misleading labels

LESS SICK DAYS!

These proven techniques STRENGTHENS YOUR IMMUNE SYSTEM! You and your family will get sick less, less work and school days missed, and less medical bills

IMPROVE MEMORY AND BEHAVIOR!

Food directly impacts your brain! Learn which foods to eat and avoid to improve yours and your kid's memory, energy, focus, and behavior

YOUR BODY MAKES ITS OWN MEDICINE!

Tap into your body's own "pharmacy" to decrease risk of nutrition-related diseases in children and adults such as ADHD, allergies, rashes, diabetes, high blood pressure, arthritis, and more!

*This is not a weight loss journal, but when you start eating cleaner, you reset your metabolism, your body begins to heal itself, and you will reach your ideal weight for your body size

HEALTHY HABITS CHANGE LIVES

Hi, I'm Perry the Penguin! Find me throughout the planner where I help you teach your kids to be an active part of this journey

Your family will be the healthiest ones on the block!

✓ Grow strong
✓ Less fatigue
✓ Less sick days
✓ Healthy brain
✓ Improved memory
✓ Improved grades in school
✓ Improved performance at work
✓ Strengthens growing hearts
✓ Sleep better
✓ Less stressed
✓ Improved creativity
✓ Less depression/anxiety

✓ Higher self-esteem
✓ Behave better
✓ Less mood swings
✓ Improves skin - acne, eczema, etc
✓ Good eyesight
✓ Promotes ideal weight for your body
✓ Learns to love healthy foods
✓ Learns their way around the supermarket

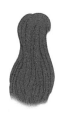

✓ More family time = improved relationships
...and so much more!

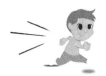

Wholistic Health

Even though the bulk of this planner is all about how to EAT CLEAN, you will learn that **everything is connected to everything**. What you eat affects your stress levels, ability to exercise, and sleep. If you're stressed, not exercising, or sleeping well, this also affects how your body digests foods and absorbs nutrients. Most of all, when you're excited to try new things and transition to a healthier lifestyle, your children pick up on that energy and become excited also. Actively including them in this journey will eventually build a special relationship that your family will remember for a lifetime.

2022

JANUARY

S	M	T	W	T	F	S
						1
2	3	4	5	6	7	8
9	10	11	12	13	14	15
16	17	18	19	20	21	22
23	24	25	26	27	28	29
30	31					

FEBRUARY

S	M	T	W	T	F	S
		1	2	3	4	5
6	7	8	9	10	11	12
13	14	15	16	17	18	19
20	21	22	23	24	25	26
27	28					

MARCH

S	M	T	W	T	F	S
		1	2	3	4	5
6	7	8	9	10	11	12
13	14	15	16	17	18	19
20	21	22	23	24	25	26
27	28	29	30	31		

APRIL

S	M	T	W	T	F	S
					1	2
3	4	5	6	7	8	9
10	11	12	13	14	15	16
17	18	19	20	21	22	23
24	25	26	27	28	29	30

MAY

S	M	T	W	T	F	S
1	2	3	4	5	6	7
8	9	10	11	12	13	14
15	16	17	18	19	20	21
22	23	24	25	26	27	28
29	30	31				

JUNE

S	M	T	W	T	F	S
			1	2	3	4
5	6	7	8	9	10	11
12	13	14	15	16	17	18
19	20	21	22	23	24	25
26	27	28	29	30		

JULY

S	M	T	W	T	F	S
					1	2
3	4	5	6	7	8	9
10	11	12	13	14	15	16
17	18	19	20	21	22	23
24	25	26	27	28	29	30
31						

AUGUST

S	M	T	W	T	F	S
	1	2	3	4	5	6
7	8	9	10	11	12	13
14	15	16	17	18	19	20
21	22	23	24	25	26	27
28	29	30	31			

SEPTEMBER

S	M	T	W	T	F	S
				1	2	3
4	5	6	7	8	9	10
11	12	13	14	15	16	17
18	19	20	21	22	23	24
25	26	27	28	29	30	

OCTOBER

S	M	T	W	T	F	S
						1
2	3	4	5	6	7	8
9	10	11	12	13	14	15
16	17	18	19	20	21	22
23	24	25	26	27	28	29
30	31					

NOVEMBER

S	M	T	W	T	F	S
		1	2	3	4	5
6	7	8	9	10	11	12
13	14	15	16	17	18	19
20	21	22	23	24	25	26
27	28	29	30			

DECEMBER

S	M	T	W	T	F	S
				1	2	3
4	5	6	7	8	9	10
11	12	13	14	15	16	17
18	19	20	21	22	23	24
25	26	27	28	29	30	31

Notes

2023

JANUARY

S	M	T	W	T	F	S
						1
2	3	4	5	6	7	8
9	10	11	12	13	14	15
16	17	18	19	20	21	22
23	24	25	26	27	28	29
30	31					

FEBRUARY

S	M	T	W	T	F	S
		1	2	3	4	5
6	7	8	9	10	11	12
13	14	15	16	17	18	19
20	21	22	23	24	25	26
27	28					

MARCH

S	M	T	W	T	F	S
			1	2	3	4	5
6	7	8	9	10	11	12
13	14	15	16	17	18	19
20	21	22	23	24	25	26
27	28	29	30	31		

APRIL

S	M	T	W	T	F	S
					1	2
3	4	5	6	7	8	9
10	11	12	13	14	15	16
17	18	19	20	21	22	23
24	25	26	27	28	29	30

MAY

S	M	T	W	T	F	S
	1	2	3	4	5	6	7
8	9	10	11	12	13	14
15	16	17	18	19	20	21
22	23	24	25	26	27	28
29	30	31				

JUNE

S	M	T	W	T	F	S
				1	2	3	4
5	6	7	8	9	10	11
12	13	14	15	16	17	18
19	20	21	22	23	24	25
26	27	28	29	30		

JULY

S	M	T	W	T	F	S
					1	2
3	4	5	6	7	8	9
10	11	12	13	14	15	16
17	18	19	20	21	22	23
24	25	26	27	28	29	30
31						

AUGUST

S	M	T	W	T	F	S
		1	2	3	4	5	6
7	8	9	10	11	12	13
14	15	16	17	18	19	20
21	22	23	24	25	26	27
28	29	30	31			

SEPTEMBER

S	M	T	W	T	F	S
				1	2	3
4	5	6	7	8	9	10
11	12	13	14	15	16	17
18	19	20	21	22	23	24
25	26	27	28	29	30	

OCTOBER

S	M	T	W	T	F	S
						1
2	3	4	5	6	7	8
9	10	11	12	13	14	15
16	17	18	19	20	21	22
23	24	25	26	27	28	29
30	31					

NOVEMBER

S	M	T	W	T	F	S
		1	2	3	4	5
6	7	8	9	10	11	12
13	14	15	16	17	18	19
20	21	22	23	24	25	26
27	28	29	30			

DECEMBER

S	M	T	W	T	F	S
				1	2	3
4	5	6	7	8	9	10
11	12	13	14	15	16	17
18	19	20	21	22	23	24
25	26	27	28	29	30	31

Notes

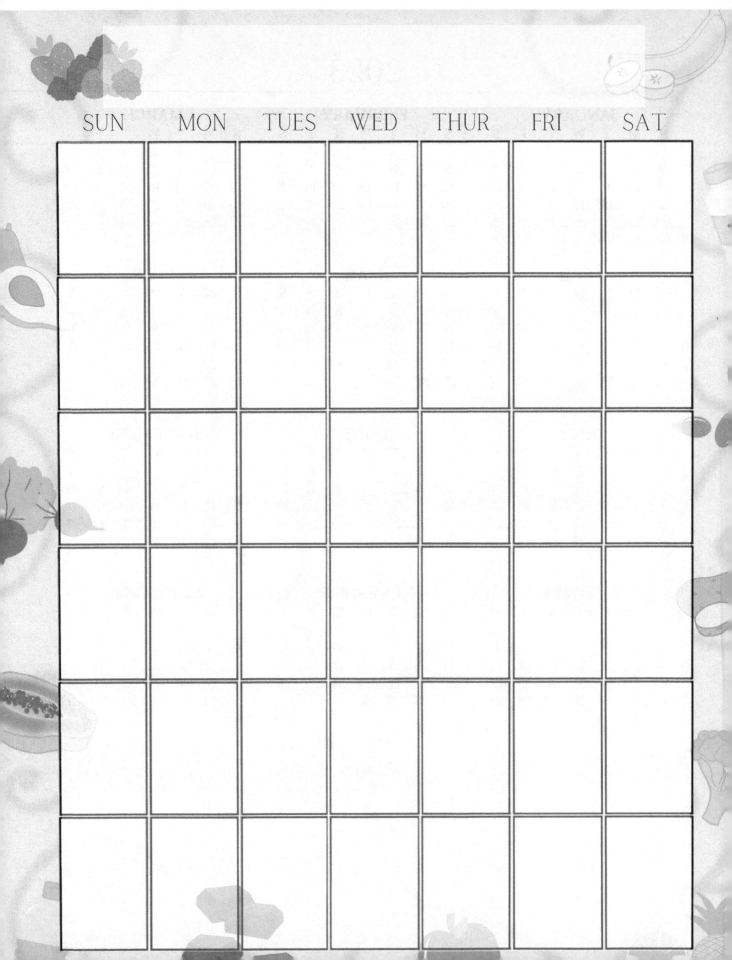

SUN	MON	TUES	WED	THUR	FRI	SAT

SUN	MON	TUES	WED	THUR	FRI	SAT

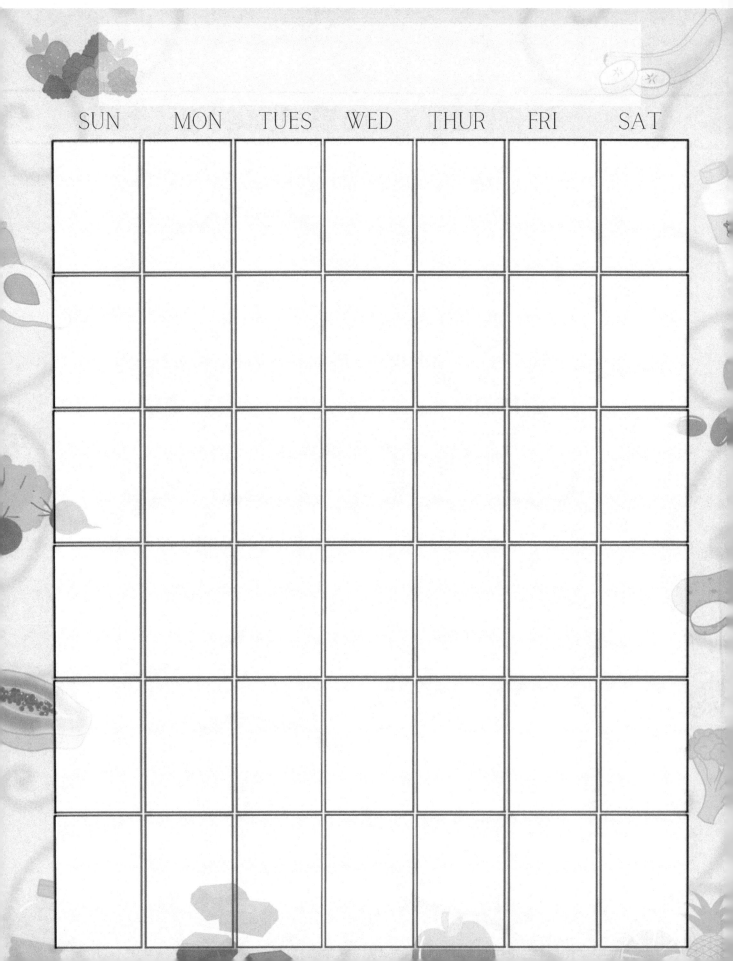

SUN	MON	TUES	WED	THUR	FRI	SAT

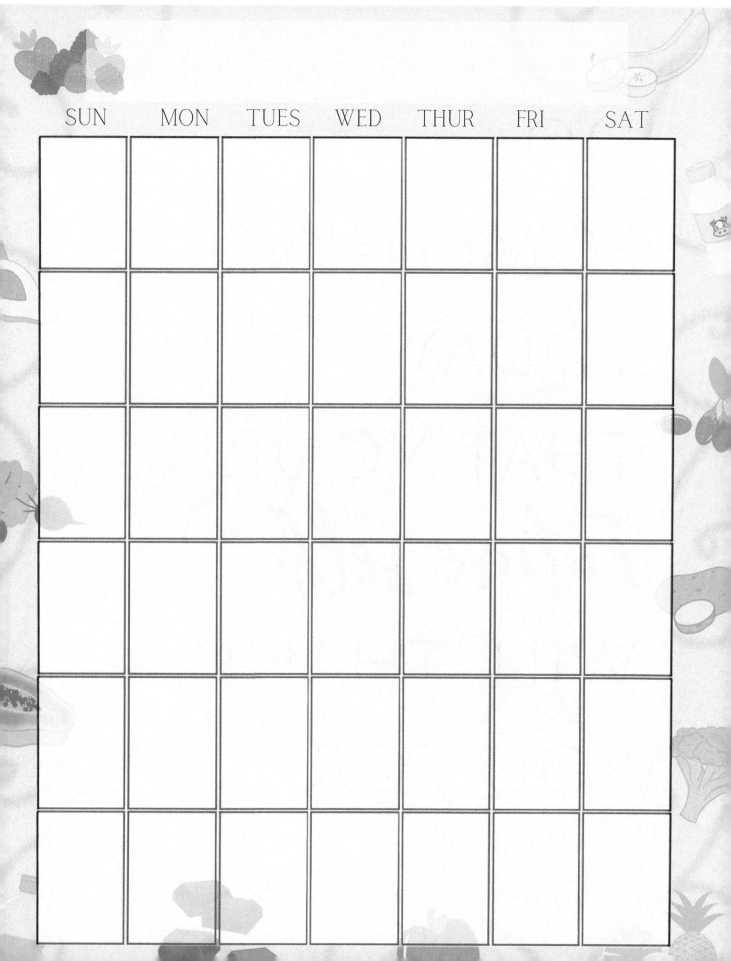

SUN	MON	TUES	WED	THUR	FRI	SAT

DO SOMETHING TODAY THAT YOUR *Future self* WILL THANK YOU FOR

PHASE ONE

ALL ABOUT NUTRITION

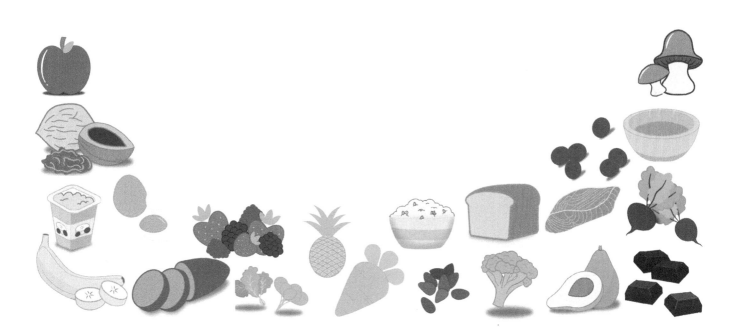

WEEK 1 CHALLENGE

☆ Get to know your planner!
   Fill in all the dates

☆ Complete your vision board

☆ Review sample page

☆ Kid's activity time

☆ Review nurse's notes

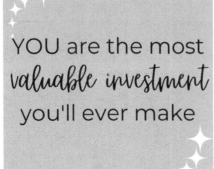

YOU are the most
valuable investment
you'll ever make

THIS WEEK'S TOP THREE

☆ _____

☆ _____

☆ _____

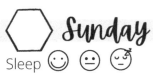

Sunday

Sleep ☺ ☺ ☺

Move your body

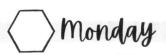

Monday

Sleep ☺ ☺ ☺

Move your body

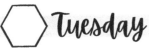

Tuesday

Sleep ☺ ☺ ☺

Move your body

Wednesday

Sleep 😊 😐 😫

Move your body

12 Thursday

Sleep 😊 😐 😫

Move your body

13 Friday

Sleep 😊 😐 😫

Move your body

14 Saturday

Sleep 😊 😐 😫

Move your body

This week, I am thankful for...

Journey to Health and Wellness

ULTIMATE GOAL

Invest in your family's health

Always be in pursuit of growth!

Love yourself enough to prioritize <u>self-care</u> and <u>gain knowledge</u> to help

TRANSFORM YOUR HABITS

Take care of your whole health by transitioning to

CLEAN EATING, MANAGING STRESS, EXERCISE, AND BETTER SLEEP

ADD LIFE TO YOUR YEARS, AND YEARS TO YOUR LIFE
- Dr. Sears

A Family's Promise

This is a WHOLE FAMILY effort. You will be each other's accountability partners.

Repeat this together. *We will support each other's journey to help stay motivated and dedicated to our commitments for a healthier and thriving family.*

I will be kind to myself

☆ ACKNOWLEDGE that your habits will not transform overnight

☆ Be BRAVE enough to take on this challenge

☆ Have CONFIDENCE in yourself that you CAN do this!

☆ Consistency is key. Be patient with yourself and your family

☆ It won't always work out perfectly, give yourself grace and keep going!

_____   _____   _____

_____   _____   _____

(Your family's signatures here)

SAMPLE PAGE

Weekly Challenges
- Color in the star when complete
- The challenges build upon the previous weeks, so keep doing them even though the week has passed!
- Most challenges will have more information on it in the next page

Weekly Affirmations/Food for thought
To maximize the effectiveness of weekly affirmations...
- WRITE IT OUT on a post-it, stick it on your habits board (see below) or on your mirror, and say it OUT LOUD every morning

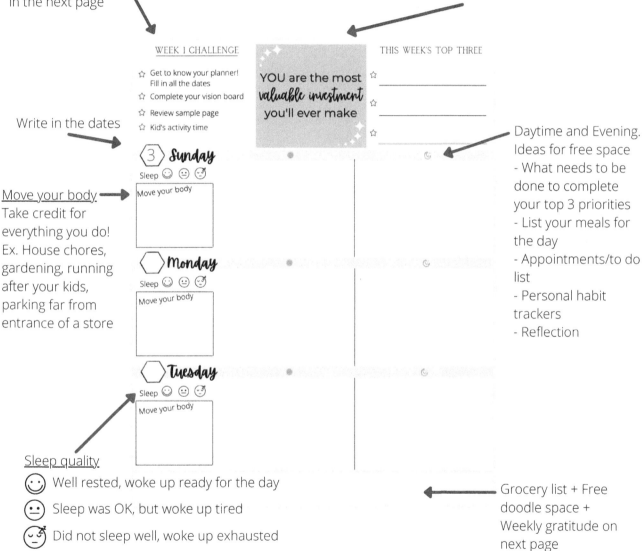

WEEK 1 CHALLENGE

☆ Get to know your planner! Fill in all the dates
☆ Complete your vision board
☆ Review sample page
☆ Kid's activity time

YOU are the most *valuable investment* you'll ever make

THIS WEEK'S TOP THREE
☆ _____
☆ _____
☆ _____

Write in the dates →

③ **Sunday**
Sleep 😊 😐 😫
Move your body

Move your body
Take credit for everything you do! Ex. House chores, gardening, running after your kids, parking far from entrance of a store

Monday
Sleep 😊 😐 😫
Move your body

Daytime and Evening. Ideas for free space
- What needs to be done to complete your top 3 priorities
- List your meals for the day
- Appointments/to do list
- Personal habit trackers
- Reflection

Tuesday
Sleep 😊 😐 😫
Move your body

Sleep quality
😊 Well rested, woke up ready for the day
😐 Sleep was OK, but woke up tired
😫 Did not sleep well, woke up exhausted

Grocery list + Free doodle space + Weekly gratitude on next page

KIDS TIME TO SHINE

This space will be used to give ideas on how to include your children. For this week, create a HEALTHY HABITS BOARD in your home (either posted on your refrigerator or a cork board) to let your family know what's happening for the week!

VISION BOARD

FIRST CHALLENGE: Draw, print, or use pictures from a magazine. Fill this page with your family's favorite things that make you happy and stay motivated. Ex. pictures of loved ones, pets, dream vacation, hobbies, favorite things, etc.

CREATIVE SPACE

You will have "off days." Look back on these pages to remind you why you started this journey!

VISION BOARD

Reaching the "ultimate goal" is not a final destination, it is something that you make the conscious decision to achieve every day in your life. You'll look back years from now and realize how far you have come!

Use this space to define what makes YOU and your family feel healthy and accomplished. What are your family's unique needs? Consider: your family's health, your children's school grades, your family's behavior, how you handle stressors - the big and small things, your productivity at home and work, your finances, etc. Clean eating can do wonders on all of this! Dig deep and DREAM BIG.

nurse's Notes
WHY IS NUTRITION SO IMPORTANT?

The World Health Organization (WHO) states that "Malnutrition, in all its forms, includes undernutrition, inadequate vitamins and minerals, overweight, obesity, and resulting diet-related non-communicable diseases." [1]

→ 38.3 million children under 5 are overweight or obese
→ Over 340 million children 5-19 are overweight or obese
→ 1.9 billion adults are overweight or obese

Global studies also report the following in children under 20 years old in 2017
→ 1.7 million incidences of cardiovascular disease
→ 28 million incidences of chronic respiratory disorders
→ 1.7 million incidences of diabetes
→ 73.7 million incidences of mental health disorders

Aren't these numbers insane?! Teaching your kids about nutrition is a priority. The habits we create about what we eat and how we eat is a LIFESTYLE we adopt as children. After all, it is one of the first things we do when we're born - EAT, right?

Raising another human being is one of the most beautiful and biggest responsibilities a parent will have in their life. You do everything for them since birth - feeding, bathing, putting them to sleep, and eventually teach them how to do it on their own. You send them to school, teach them manners and your family's values. You even teach them how to cook and clean. BUT...

→ **Don't forget to teach them how the foods we eat affect our brain, body, and behavior and how it can prevent future mental and physical disease**

Shopping, preparing, and eating the right foods are among the most important things you can teach your kids. Teach them skills and habits that will benefit them for the rest of their lives. THEY WILL THANK YOU ONE DAY!

1Malnutrition Key Facts. World Health Organization. 2021. https://www.who.int/news-room/fact-sheets/detail/malnutrition

M&M = Mindset and Motivation

This section will address different forms of self-care. Being mindful is an important skill that can be learned to help your mind, body, and soul heal.

———— Your new hobby: In pursuit of Health ————

How do you prepare for your future retirement? Most would answer putting money aside in a retirement fund, but not many would initially think to answer - preparing their bodies for good health so they can enjoy that retirement. Most don't appreciate their health until it starts to decline. Learn to decrease your risk of spending your time and retirement money at frequent doctor's appointments, having little energy, and being unable to do the things you love due to aging or chronic condition.

Invest in your health now to prepare for a stronger future, it's never too late!

Your journey to health and wellness will become a lifelong hobby. Become obsessed and make it a family project! When you're ready to put your mental, physical, and spiritual needs above everything else, you will find that life will fall into place better than you believed it could be. Taking care of yourself is an act of **self-love**, which teaches your family that it is OK to do that for themselves as well. Challenging yourself in this lifelong hobby is a great way for you and your family to grow together and create habits that'll serve you for generations. Trying new foods and activities with your family will also strengthen your minds and bodies to keep them sharp!

MAKE A PLAN WRITE out your daily affirmations on a post-it. Where is the best place to stick it so that you and your family can repeat it OUT LOUD every morning?

Promise to myself: _____

☆ Set aside 5-10 minutes twice
a week to fill out your journal
☐ ☐ ☐ ☐ ☐ ☐ ☐

☆ Start reading the nutrition
label of everything you eat
☐ ☐ ☐ ☐ ☐ ☐ ☐

☆ Kid's time to shine activity

Eating healthy
is how I show
I love my body

THIS WEEK'S TOP THREE

☆ _____

☆ _____

☆ _____

15 Sunday

Sleep 😊 😐 😴

Move your body

16 Monday

Sleep 😊 😐 😴

Move your body

17 Tuesday

Sleep 😊 😐 😴

Move your body

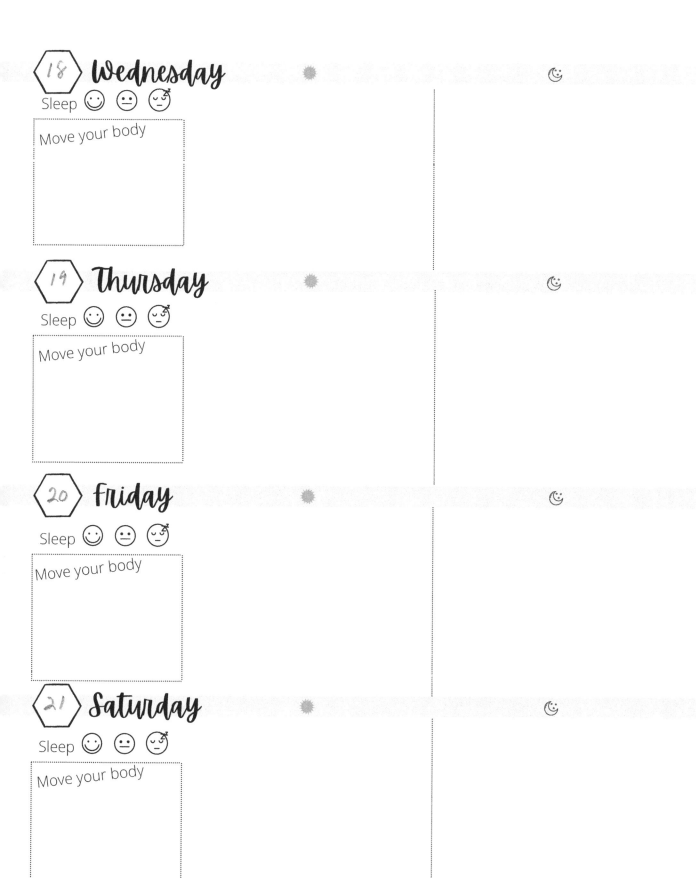

⬡ 18 Wednesday

Sleep 🙂 😐 😴

Move your body

⬡ 19 Thursday

Sleep 🙂 😐 😴

Move your body

⬡ 20 Friday

Sleep 🙂 😐 😴

Move your body

⬡ 21 Saturday

Sleep 🙂 😐 😴

Move your body

Something I handled well...

M&M MOMENT

Challenge: *Set aside at least 5-10 minutes each week to fill out your journal*

The first 7 days of committing to anything new is always the hardest, but hang in there, it does get easier! Creating a new habit is like working out a muscle, it'll get stronger the more you practice. Planning to set aside time to work on yourself in advance helps you to set your intentions for the week. This is especially important because of how busy we can get. But a part of self-care is taking a moment to gather your thoughts, reflect on your day and appreciate the good and bad that is creating the person you are. **Don't let life pass you by!**

For example, my evening routine consists of spending 10 minutes reflecting on my day to see if I completed the things I said I would, filling out my gratitude moment, and then roughly planning out my next day. So yes, I fill out the next day's "daytime entry" already. Here is an example...

WEEK 2 CHALLENGE

☆ Set aside 5-10 minutes twice each week to fill out your journal
☐ ☐ ☐ ☐ ☐ ☐ ☐

☆ Start reading the nutrition label of everything you eat
☐ ☐ ☐ ☐ ☐ ☐ ☐

☆ Kid's time to shine activity

⬡ **Sunday**

Sleep ☺ ☺ ☺

Move your body

Eating healthy is how I show *I love my body*

THIS WEEK'S TOP THREE

☆ Complete assignment due this week for school by Wednesday

☆ Prepare preschool supplies for teachers by Thursday

☆ Complete this week's challenge on Saturday during family time

☐ Wake up early to work on assignment before the kids wake up. max 2 hours
☐ Breakfast: Sweet potato hash and eggs
☐ Spend 30 min at the park
☐ Shop for preschool supplies
☐ lunch: protein smoothie bowls
☐ Quiet play time 15-2 hours
☐ Prepare dinner: brown rice, steamed veggies and salmon

Do what works for you! This can be done on your own or with your family. 5 minutes in the morning and 5 minutes at night, or all 10 minutes in the evening. Good luck!

MAKE A PLAN Which day and what time will I be filling out this journal?

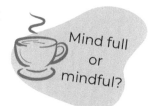
Mind full or mindful?

Promise to myself: _____

_____

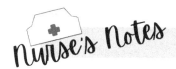

NUTRITION LABEL

Challenge: *Start reading the nutrition label of everything you eat.*

Begin reading the nutrition label of every food item in your pantry and before you buy anything new. In the next several weeks, you'll learn the recommended daily nutrients for yourself and your growing children to improve your attitude, energy levels, memory and prevent diseases!

Start at the Top

Servings Per Container:
- Total number of servings in the entire package or container

Serving Size:
- The serving size is a guide, NOT the recommendation of how much to eat

Eat less ...
- Fat
- Cholesterol
- Sodium
- Sugars

Eat more ...
- Dietary Fiber
- Protein

% Daily Value
- Based on a 2000 calorie per day diet
- Low = 5% Daily Value or less per serving of a nutrient
- High = 20% Daily Value or more of a nutrient

Nutrition Facts
about 12 servings per container
Serving size 3 cookies (34g)

Amount per serving
Calories 160

	% Daily Value*
Total Fat 7g	9%
Saturated Fat 2g	10%
Trans Fat 0g	
Cholesterol 0mg	0%
Sodium 135mg	6%
Total Carbohydrate 25g	9%
Dietary Fiber less than 1g	2%
Total Sugars 14g	
Includes 14g Added Sugars	28%
Protein 1g	
Vitamin D 0mcg	0%
Calcium 10mg	0%
Iron 1.4mg	8%
Potassium 50mg	0%

* The % Daily Value (DV) tells you how much a nutrient in a serving of food contributes to a daily diet. 2,000 calories a day is used for general nutrition advice.

When going through your pantry, ask...

☐ Is it high in protein?

☐ Is it high in fiber?

☐ Is it low in added sugars?

*These numbers are based on where you're currently at. Always work towards being better than yesterday!

KID'S TIME TO SHINE

Teach your kids how to read nutrition labels around the home at first, then at the stores! Make it a game - who can pick out a snack with the least sugar?

POP QUIZ

1 serving of cookies = 3 cookies

1. If I ate 6 cookies, how many servings did I eat? _____

2. How many total calories was my 6 cookies? _____

3. How many total grams of sugars did I eat? _____

4. How much of my daily value in sugar did I eat? _____

Answers: 1. 2 2. 160x2=320 calories 3. 14x2=28 g sugar 4. 28x2=56% DVi

WEEK 3 CHALLENGE

☆ Start reading the ingredient's label on everything you eat

☐ ☐ ☐ ☐ ☐ ☐ ☐

☆ Pantry scavenger hunt - Watch out for the "forbidden four"

☆ Kid's time to shine activity

Excuses are the enemy of *progress*

THIS WEEK'S TOP THREE

☆ _____

☆ _____

☆ _____

⬡ Sunday

Sleep ☺ 😐 😴

Move your body

⬡ Monday

Sleep ☺ 😐 😴

Move your body

⬡ Tuesday

Sleep ☺ 😐 😴

Move your body

Wednesday

Sleep 🙂 😐 😴

Move your body

Thursday

Sleep 🙂 😐 😴

Move your body

Friday

Sleep 🙂 😐 😴

Move your body

Saturday

Sleep 🙂 😐 😴

Move your body

A person I appreciated...

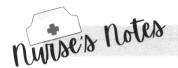

INGREDIENT'S LIST

Challenge: *Start to read the ingredient's label on everything you eat*

After reading through the Nutrition Facts, the next step is to read through the ingredients list. This is the MOST IMPORTANT part of a nutrition label. When going through your pantry or before purchasing anything new, ask these questions...

☐ Is the list short or long?

☐ Which ingredients are listed first?

☐ Can you pronounce most of the words?

☐ Does it include the "forbidden four?"

Look for:

- Short list of ingredients (10 or less is best)
- Whole foods (WHOLE grain), organic, foods you recognize, etc
- *First* in the list means *most* in the food
- Words you can pronounce

Example: Ingredients List From a Store Bought Granola

Dates, Organic Bananas, Walnuts, Sunflower Seeds, Pumpkin Seeds, Dry Roasted Cashews (Cashews, Sea Salt), Pecans, Cinnamon, Vanilla Bean

Avoid:

✗ Long list of ingredients (10 or more)

✗ "Forbidden Four" → High fructose corn syrup, hydrogenated oil, artificial sugars, and colors

✗ Food additives, chemicals or foods you don't recognize

Example: Ingredients List From a Popular Breakfast Pastry

Enriched flour (wheat flour, niacin, reduced iron, vitamin B1 (thiamin moninitrate), vitamin B2 (riboflavin), folic acid, corny syrup, high fructose corn syrup, soybean and palm oil, (with TBHQ for freshness), sugar, dextrose, contains 2% or less of modified corn starch, salt, cornstarch, cream, leavening (baking soda, sodium acid pyrophosphate, monocalcium phosphate), strawberry powder, hydrogenated palm kernal oil, soy lecithin, gelatin, color added, natural and artificial flavors, xanthan gum, DATEM, strawberry juice concentrate, red 40, yellow 5, yellow 6, blue 1, carnauba wax, blue 2

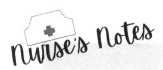

FORBIDDEN FOUR

Challenge: *Watch out for the "forbidden four"*

When reading the ingredients list, keep in mind that some chemicals can have **multiple names**

Food Additive	Also known as	Possible Health Effects
High Fructose Corn Syrup	Fructose syrup, corn syrup, glucose syrup	Weight gain, diabetes, heart disease, and inflammation
Trans Fat	Hydrogenated vegetable oil, shortening	Premature heart attacks, heart disease, increase blood sugar and inflammation
Artificial Sweeteners	Aspartame, sucralose, acesulfame potassium, saccharin	Risk of cancer, diabetes, obesity, negative impact on the gut microbiome
Artificial Colorings	Yellow 5, Red 40, Blue 1, etc.	Cause hyperactivity in some children, allergy-like reactions and risk of cancer

Chemical Cuisine. Center for Science in the Public. Interest.https://www.cspinet.org/eating-healthy/chemical-cuisine

Go through your pantry. Write down the foods that contain the "forbidden four" ingredients. Bonus: Apply red stickers on each item to help kids visualize which foods to not eat every day

☐ _____

☐ _____

☐ _____

☐ _____

☐ _____

Did you know?

Even if the package says ZERO TRANS FAT, the food is legally still able to contain half a gram of trans fat. This is the reason why checking the ingredients label is most important and reliable!

MAKE A PLAN

Decrease your intake. Start small, if you eat this daily, aim for every other day and decrease over time. Categorize your pantry, separating these foods on another shelf. There is usually a version of your favorite foods without the "forbidden four!" Look for one and post it in our FB group to share or find out suggestions

Promise to myself: _____

_____

WEEK 4 CHALLENGE

☆ Drink enough water for your body weight

☐ ☐ ☐ ☐ ☐ ☐ ☐

☆ Kid's time to shine activity

☆ Turn off all distractions during meal times (TV/radio/phones)

☐ ☐ ☐ ☐ ☐ ☐ ☐

I will not sacrifice my *Nutrition and Health* for convenience

THIS WEEK'S TOP THREE

☆ _____

☆ _____

☆ _____

Sunday

Sleep ☺ 😐 😣

Move your body

Monday

Sleep ☺ 😐 😣

Move your body

Tuesday

Sleep ☺ 😐 😣

Move your body

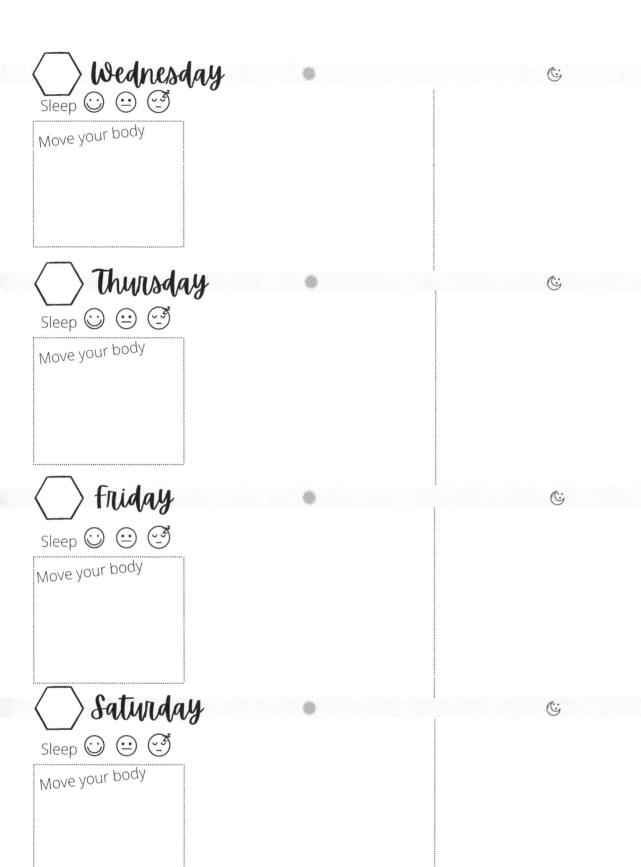

Wednesday

Sleep 😊 😐 😫

Move your body

Thursday

Sleep 😊 😐 😫

Move your body

Friday

Sleep 😊 😐 😫

Move your body

Saturday

Sleep 😊 😐 😫

Move your body

Something new I learned...

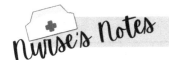

Challenge: *Drink enough water for YOUR body weight*

—Why is water so important? ——————————

- **Water prevents you from overeating**. Sometimes when we think we're hungry, we're really thirsty! Drink a cup of water before each meal and another cup before reaching for a snack
- **The brain is 70-75% water**. When it doesn't get enough water, it can't function effectively
- **Your muscles are 70-75% water**. When the muscles don't get enough water, it's dehydrated and gets tired easily
- **Water cleanses the body**. Your body needs water to help your kidneys clean out the toxins and waste products from the body
- **Water helps you heal when sick**. Drinking lots of water keeps your airways from drying out and helps loosen thick secretions. This helps you cough out germs more effectively. Water will also keep your body cool and hydrated if you're having fevers and sweats

———————— How much should you drink? ——

	CHILDREN	ADULTS
NEED	1 oz water per 1 pound of weight	1/2 oz water per 1 pound of weight
EXAMPLE 1 standard water bottle = 16.9 oz	50lb child needs 50oz of water 3 water bottles	150lb adult needs 75 oz of water 4.5 water bottles

*Children need more water per lb of weight because their little bodies use up more water and electrolytes faster than adults

KID'S TIME TO SHINE

 Purchase new water bottles for the family! Let your kids pick their own water bottles and decorate them with waterproof stickers for fun. Buy number stickers so you can put the number of times it needs to be refilled in a day to fulfill their unique needs. Check out our Etsy store - www.shophealthyliving.etsy.com for ideas!

M&M MOMENT

Challenge: *Turn off all distractions during mealtimes (TV/radio/phones)*

Have you ever eaten a whole bag of popcorn or chips while watching a movie? You get to the bottom and wondered where did all the food go? Watching TV or using your devices during meal times is a distraction and can mask our body's cues that tell you whether you're full or still hungry.

Your body gives you the opportunity to do the things you love, like play with your children, and work to provide for your family. Thank your bodies by listening to their cues and fueling them with the right nutrients. The FIRST step in doing this is putting away your devices, truly enjoying the food you eat, and listening to your body's cues.

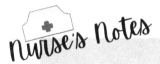

HARM REDUCTION

In public health, harm reduction is defined as "a set of practical strategies and ideas aimed at reducing negative consequences associated with drug use."[1] Note the word - REDUCING... Their goal is not to STOP drug use, but to help those who use, reduce the harmful effects associated with drugs. **WHAT!**

Why am I talking about this? Because I want you to recognize that an unhealthy relationship with food exists and is a REAL problem - **overeating the wrong foods and not eating enough of the right foods**. This leads to obesity, heart disease, diabetes, Alzheimer's, you name it...

My goal is NOT to stop you from eating the "fun" unhealthy foods, but instead to educate you on its effects. There's a time and place to eat anything you want, so you don't feel restricted. Knowing this, we can come up with a plan to safely include these foods in your diet, while still improving and maintaining your health! This supports the non-diet and abundance mindset. You can still have your cake, and eat it too!

1 Harm Reduction. National Harm Reduction Coalition. 2021. https://harmreduction.org/about-us/principles-of-harm-reduction/

MONTHLY REFLECTION

Use this time to review your vision board and update as needed!

☆ A moment I can't forget...

☆ The hardest thing about this past month was...

☆ We got through the hardest times together by...

☆ I am so proud of...

☆ Best meal I thouroughly enjoyed:

☆ The funniest thing that happened was...

KID'S TIME TO SHINE

Space for your kids to write or draw what they enjoyed the most this last month

MONTHLY HABIT TRACKER

Print one out for each family member & post it on your family board.
Which habits do you want to concentrate on to make sure your family is continuing
it daily? Color it in after completing it & celebrate every day's win! 1 symbol = 1 day.

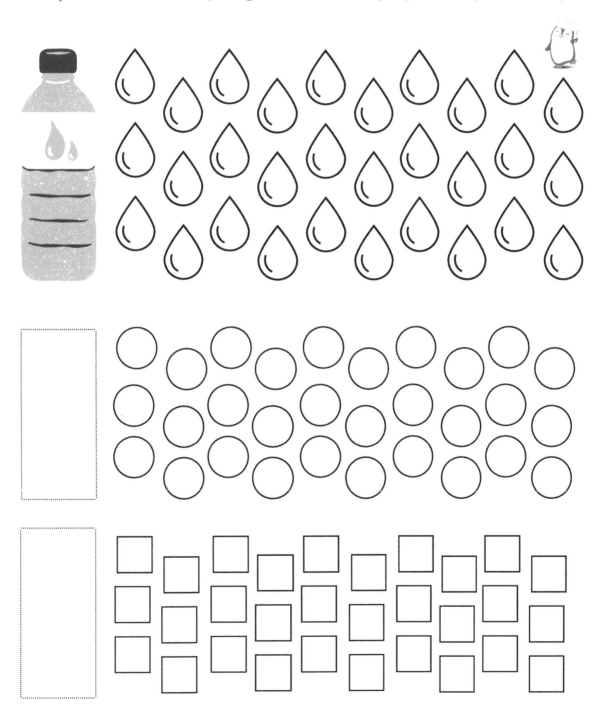

☆ Don't drink your calories! No juices, electrolyte waters or sodas this week!

☐ ☐ ☐ ☐ ☐ ☐ ☐

☆ Review nurse's notes

☆ Fill out monthly habit tracker

Nothing will work *Unless you do*

- Maya Angelou

THIS WEEK'S TOP THREE

☆ _____

☆ _____

☆ _____

Sunday

Sleep 🙂 😐 😴

Move your body

Monday

Sleep 🙂 😐 😴

Move your body

Tuesday

Sleep 🙂 😐 😴

Move your body

Wednesday

Sleep ☺ 😐 😔

Move your body

Thursday

Sleep ☺ 😐 😔

Move your body

Friday

Sleep ☺ 😐 😔

Move your body

Saturday

Sleep ☺ 😐 😔

Move your body

I am proud of myself for...

Challenge: *Don't drink your calories! No juices, electrolyte waters or sodas this week!*

- Check the ingredient's label of your juices. Especially labels that say "zero sugar" or "low sugar," they may contain other harmful additives in your "juice" including the forbidden four!

Ingredients from a popular zero calorie fruit punch

- Pure filtered water, lemon juice from concentrate, less than 2% of: grape and pineapple juices from concentrate, natural flavors, citric acid, vitamin c, aspartame, acesulfame potassium, grape skin extract.

If you need flavored drinks, try these REAL FOOD alternatives (not the "natural flavor" stuff - what does that really mean?!)

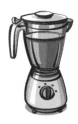

- When you have a blender, anything is possible!
- Cut up an apple, remove seeds, and blend it with water for all-natural APPLE JUICE. Including the skin adds fiber to your apple juice!
- Try something more adventurous like this Strawberry Agua Fresca! Blend together 1 cup of strawberries, 2 mint leaves, a squeeze of lime juice, and water. Add a bit of honey or coconut sugar for sweetness

- If blending is not your thing, simply adding cut fruits and veggies are amazing too!

- My favorite: a handful of sliced cucumbers, a couple of mint leaves, and fresh strawberries. Combine with water in a large pitcher. Let it sit for a few hours until all the flavors have infused into the water. It's so refreshing, enjoy!

Freeze into popsicles or your kid's favorite shaped silicone molds!

FB POST What's your favorite ingredients to make "flavored water?

THE TRUTH ABOUT "ELECTROLYTES WATER"

Drinks that have added electrolytes or vitamins are marketed as "good for you." Some will insist it gives you energy, focus better, or re-hydrate you on a hot day. But, let's look at the facts....

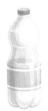

Popular zero-calorie
sports drink
for hydration

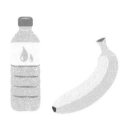

Nutrition Facts

About 2.5 servings per container
Serving size   12 fl oz (360mL)

Calories		Per Container **10**
		% DV*
Total fat	0g	0%
Sodium	380mg	16%
Total Carb.	2g	1%
Total Sugars	0g	
Incl. Added Sugars	0g	0%
Protein	0g	
Potassium	110mg	2%

- Water, citric acid, natural flavor, sodium citrate, salt, monopotassium phosphate, modified food starch, mixed triglycerides, sucralose, glycerol ester of rosin, acesulfame potassium

Nutrition Facts

Serving size
1 medium banana (118g)

Calories		Per Container **105**
		% DV*
Total fat	0.4g	1%
Sodium	2mg	0%
Total Carb.	27g	9%
Dietary Fiber	3g	12%
Sugars	14g	
Protein	1g	
Potassium	358g	8%
Vitamin A		2%
Vitamin C		17%
Calcium		1%
Iron		2%

A banana still has more potassium than THREE bottles of sports drink!

Contains more than one of the "forbidden four" ingredients

**In conclusion, drinking a bottle of water and eating a banana will offer more hydration and electrolyte replacement than a sports drink!
- Another great natural alternative? Coconut water and watermelon water**

MAKE A PLAN

If you drink these, make a plan to decrease your intake. Start small, if you drink this daily, aim for every other day and decrease over time

Promise to myself: _____

_____

WEEK 6 CHALLENGE

☆ Watch your portions! Eat only until you are not hungry

☐ ☐ ☐ ☐ ☐ ☐ ☐

☆ Are you still drinking all your water?

☐ ☐ ☐ ☐ ☐ ☐ ☐

☆ Kid's time to shine activity

You are never too old to set another goal or *Dream a new dream*

- C.S. Lewis

THIS WEEK'S TOP THREE

☆ _____

☆ _____

☆ _____

Sunday

Sleep 😊 😐 😴

Move your body

Monday

Sleep 😊 😐 😴

Move your body

Tuesday

Sleep 😊 😐 😴

Move your body

⬡ Wednesday

Sleep 🙂 😐 😫

Move your body

⬡ Thursday

Sleep 🙂 😐 😫

Move your body

⬡ Friday

Sleep 🙂 😐 😫

Move your body

⬡ Saturday

Sleep 🙂 😐 😫

Move your body

Something that brought me joy this week...

M&M MOMENT

Challenge: *Watch your portions. Give yourself a chance to listen to your body and learn your hunger cues*

—Portion Control—

You have the power to make this lifestyle choice with every meal

- **Use smaller plates**

- **Avoid the need to "clean your plate."** Decide when to stop eating based on how your stomach feels, not how much food is left on the plate. Those last few bites are better in the trash than in your stomach! Once your stomach stretches, it sends a signal to your brain to say it's full. Ignoring this signal multiple times could make it difficult to recognize it one day, leading to chronic overeating

- **Snack on fresh fruits or cut vegetables** before and/or after eating your meals. This can help meet your daily servings of fruits and vegetables

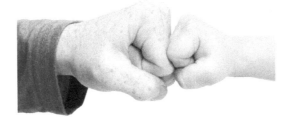

Adult vs. Child Portions

- Your stomach is the size of your fist. Use this to determine the size of your meals and snacks. Your stomach can stretch to accommodate more food. But once it starts to stretch, it sends a signal to our brain that tells us to stop. Try to pay close attention to that signal!

KID'S TIME TO SHINE

Let your children serve themselves! Empower them to put all their favorite fixings on their plates in the portions they desire, while still encouraging them to try new food items. This helps them be more mindful about their portions.

M&M MOMENT

Grazing

Your body is smart and it's your job to listen to it

- Infants and babies breastfeed or bottlefeed every 2-3 hours and toddlers often need snacks throughout the day

- Some adults may feel better eating several small meals, and some prefer a traditional breakfast, lunch, and dinner plus snacks in between, or at bedtime

- See which works out for your lifestyle. Whatever you do, don't skip meals!

*If you "diet" frequently, sometimes you lose the ability to listen to your hunger cues. Do NOT wait until you're hungry to eat! Your body NEEDS nutrients to heal, so train it to eat portioned meals throughout the day. If you skip meals, this increases your stress hormone and tells your body to store the food as fat, instead of using the nutrients to repair and nourish your body. Eating regularly will help stabilize your metabolism.

Water

MAKE A PLAN

Sometimes when you think you're hungry, you're really thirsty! Are you able to drink the amount of water you need for your body weight? Let's create rules to make sure this is happening. Pick a scenario that you do daily and PLAN when you will drink water.

Promise to myself I will keep a water bottle with me at all times and drink water....

☐ Every time I get up or sit back down   ☐ Before going to bed

☐ After I use the restroom   ☐ As I am preparing my meals

☐ Shortly after waking up   ☐ After finishing my meal

☐ _____   ☐ _____

☐ _____   ☐ _____

☆ Slow down while you eat!

☐ ☐ ☐ ☐ ☐ ☐ ☐

☆ Learn to use the hunger scale

☐ ☐ ☐ ☐ ☐ ☐ ☐

☆ Kid's time to shine activity

don't focus on
how much you eat
focus on
what you eat

☆ _____

☆ _____

☆ _____

⬡ **Sunday**

Sleep ☺ 😐 😴

Move your body

⬡ **Monday**

Sleep ☺ 😐 😴

Move your body

⬡ **Tuesday**

Sleep ☺ 😐 😴

Move your body

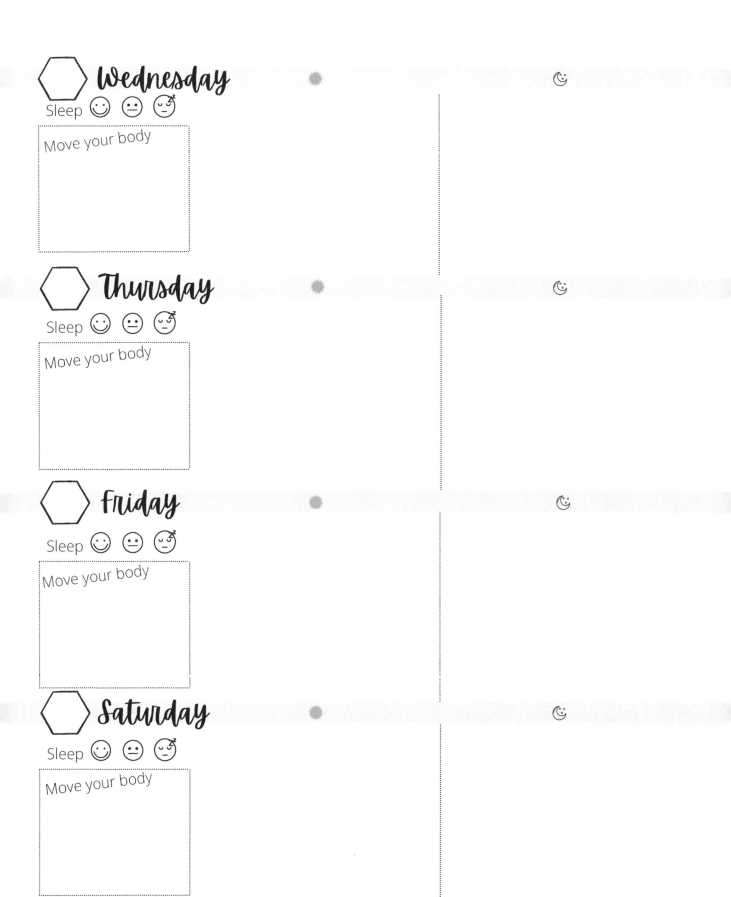

Wednesday

Sleep 🙂 😐 😴

Move your body

Thursday

Sleep 🙂 😐 😴

Move your body

Friday

Sleep 🙂 😐 😴

Move your body

Saturday

Sleep 🙂 😐 😴

Move your body

Share a favorite memory that always make you smile...

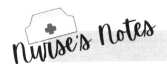

M&M MOMENT

Challenge: *Slow down while you eat!*

── Slow Down ──

- **Use all five senses to appreciate your food**. Seriously! Your brain and digestive system are intimately connected. You need BOTH of these major systems ready for it to digest food and absorb nutrients efficiently.

> **SMELL** is the first and most powerful sense that tells your brain it is time to eat. Pay attention and **hear** the foods being prepared to tell your body it is almost time. **Look** at your food, feel the texture of your food as it enters your mouth, and **taste** the flavors. **Chew** slowly until your food is close to liquid, don't swallow large chunks of food! Chewing your food slowly and completely gives your brain time to anticipate the next steps so that it can release the right enzymes and allow the stomach and intestines to absorb nutrients more efficiently. It also increases satiety and decreases the risk of overeating.

── Tips ──

- Spend the first several minutes of each meal talking about the food! Have each family member guess the ingredients using taste, texture, or by looking at it. This will also teach them to appreciate the time and love it takes for parents (or the restaurant) put into preparing a meal!

- Play a game with young children. Have them count how many times they chew each bite to encourage them to slow down and chew more

- Drink water after every few bites

- Make mealtimes a social occasion. Try to have at least one meal together as a family. This is a great time to connect and build a positive influence with your children. Talk about the highs and lows in your day. Talking during a meal helps everyone take their time eating and the opportunity to realize their hunger cues

HUNGER SCALE

- Use this chart to help understand your hunger cues

- Don't allow yourself to get past hungry into starving, and only eat until you're satisfied

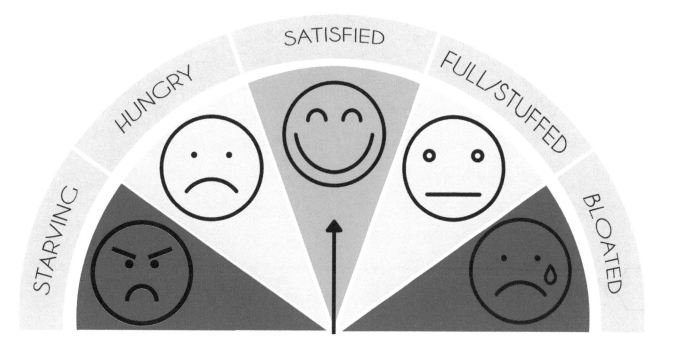

KID'S TIME TO SHINE

Make a copy of this scale and post it on your Healthy Habits board or refrigerator as a constant reminder! Kids love visuals and seeing this could help them understand their own hunger cues.

☆ Create your mental "tool belt"

☆ Review Nurse's Notes:
  Gratitude

☆ Kid's time to shine activity

The greatest gift you
can give your family
and the world is a
healthy you

- Joyce Meyer

☆ _____

☆ _____

☆ _____

Sunday

Sleep 😊 😐 😴

Move your body

Monday

Sleep 😊 😐 😴

Move your body

Tuesday

Sleep 😊 😐 😴

Move your body

Wednesday

Sleep 🙂 😐 😴

Move your body

Thursday

Sleep 🙂 😐 😴

Move your body

Friday

Sleep 🙂 😐 😴

Move your body

Saturday

Sleep 🙂 😐 😴

Move your body

I am thankful for...

Challenge: *Create your mental "tool belt" to help manage those tough times*

If you or your children are having a tough time responding to those who question your new lifestyle changes (or you're questioning yourself!), it is important to have a fully stocked tool belt to help you manage those tough times under peer pressure.

 BE PROUD OF YOURSELF.

Seriously. It takes a lot of courage to make any lifestyle changes and you shouldn't be ashamed of yourself. For example, don't let others pressure you into that second pint of beer when you only PLANNED to have one! When you say no to something, say it with conviction and feel EMPOWERED you had the strength to do so, don't feel sorry for yourself or feel restricted!

Use the WE principle.

When addressing new lifestyle changes, you don't have to feel alone! Explain that WE as a family are working together to prevent chronic diseases or focus better on work/school. This works especially great for children when trying to explain certain boundaries. Instead of saying "Put away your phones and turn off the TV while we eat dinner," say "We eat together as a family without distractions from our phones and TV."

 LOVE YOURSELF. YOU DESERVE IT.

You're doing this because it will make you FEEL good. Remember the promises you made to yourself during your first week? Review that. Keep your promises to yourself and teach your kids the power of believing in yourself knowing you can do anything you put your mind to.

MAKE A PLAN
Write what you would tell yourself and others on days that you are having a tough time following through with your vision... What is your MANTRA?

Promise to myself:_____

_____

Notes to self

Every small decision I make today makes a big difference in tomorrow. Working towards a healthy and happy body is an ongoing goal. I'm in this for the long run!	It is so difficult to be consistent EVERY DAY. I will practice unconditional forgiveness for myself the entire journey.	Feeding my children healthy meals now will condition their preferences for healthy meals in the future.

gratitude

Are you doing your weekly gratitude? Consciously making an effort to look at the bright side of life has many benefits for our mental health. Designate a time each day to reflect on your day and think of anything that made you smile. Sharing with your family is the best way!

Benefits

- Allows you to focus on the present
- Increases bonding and positive mood
- Improves satisfaction with life
- You're more forgiving

- Improves sleep
- Improves immune system
- More resistant to stress
- Blocks negative emotions

KID'S TIME TO SHINE

Teach your kids the significance of pointing out the good things that happen. Create a gratitude jar - either for the whole family or for each individual. Prepare a small notepad and pen that stays next to the jar. Write down the date and something special - big or small. Try to do this most days of the week. At the end of the year for Thanksgiving or New Years, review all the notes in there!

MONTHLY REFLECTION

Use this time to review your vision board and update as needed!

☆ What were your family's biggest accomplishments?

☆ What were your biggest fears/stressors?

☆ How did you or do you plan on overcoming those fears/stressors?

☆ Have you noticed any changes in your family, such as behavior, symptoms or etc.?

☆ I am so proud of...

☆ Best meal I thouroughly enjoyed:

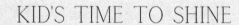

KID'S TIME TO SHINE

Space for your kids to write or draw what they enjoyed the most this last month

MONTHLY HABIT TRACKER

Print one out for each family member & post it on your family board! Track the habits you are concentrating on. Color it in after completing it and celebrate every day's win! 1 symbol = 1 day.

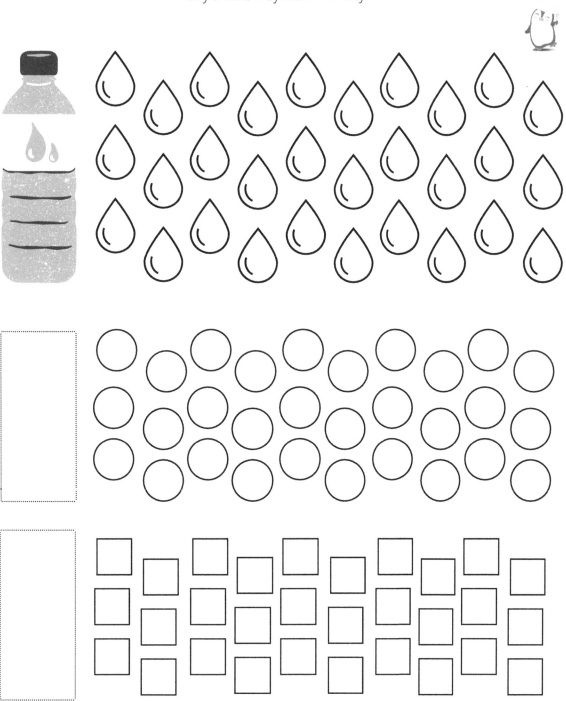

WEEK 9 CHALLENGE

☆ Pick one new habit from previous weeks you still need work on

☐ ☐ ☐ ☐ ☐ ☐ ☐

☆ Send a message to someone each day to express your gratitude.

☐ ☐ ☐ ☐ ☐ ☐ ☐

EVEN THE SMALLEST SHIFT IN PERSPECTIVE CAN BRING ABOUT THE GREATEST HEALING

— JOSHUA KAI

THIS WEEK'S TOP THREE

☆ _____

☆ _____

☆ _____

⬡ **Sunday**

Sleep 🙂 😐 😫

Move your body

⬡ **Monday**

Sleep 🙂 😐 😫

Move your body

⬡ **Tuesday**

Sleep 🙂 😐 😫

Move your body

⬡ *Wednesday*

Sleep 🙂 😐 😴

Move your body

⬡ *Thursday*

Sleep 🙂 😐 😴

Move your body

⬡ *Friday*

Sleep 🙂 😐 😴

Move your body

⬡ *Saturday*

Sleep 🙂 😐 😴

Move your body

Something I handled well...

WEEK 10 CHALLENGE

☆ Create a list of meals and snacks for your family
☐ ☐ ☐ ☐ ☐ ☐ ☐

☆ Set a good example for change by staying positive. Don't use negative self-talk, the kids are listening!
☐ ☐ ☐ ☐ ☐ ☐ ☐

Never give up on *you*

THIS WEEK'S TOP THREE

☆ _____

☆ _____

☆ _____

⬡ Sunday

Sleep ☺ 😐 😴

Move your body

⬡ Monday

Sleep ☺ 😐 😴

Move your body

⬡ Tuesday

Sleep ☺ 😐 😴

Move your body

Wednesday

Sleep ☺ 😐 😫

Move your body

Thursday

Sleep ☺ 😐 😫

Move your body

Friday

Sleep ☺ 😐 😫

Move your body

Saturday

Sleep ☺ 😐 😫

Move your body

A person I appreciated...

M&M MOMENT: FAMILY MEAL PLAN

Challenge: *Create a list of the most common meals and snacks your family eats. Include your favorite foods you wish you would eat more often!*

Creating a visual list is a great tool to analyze your overall food intake and helps **decrease decision fatigue** when it comes to meal planning.

The biggest reasons we resort to eating junk food are...
we're in a hurry and/or we're already hungry

These two are dangerous when felt at the same time because you won't be able to make a proper decision nor have the energy to prepare a healthier meal. Unfortunately, it can be difficult to avoid this situation. What's the solution? PREPARE for these moments.

—————— Family Meal Plan Tips ——————

→ Write down foods your family currently eats AND what you wish to eat more of

→ **Breakfasts**: Categorize breakfasts based on preparation time. Ex. We only make these on the weekends vs. these are quick to prepare before work/school. *Star the ones that are easiest and on the go!

→ **Snacks**: Categorize snacks that are OK to eat anytime vs snacks that are meant for once in a while. Ex. I'll only buy one family-size bag of chips to enjoy during movie nights twice a month, but I'll have healthy granola bars and apples available at all times

→ **Must have fast foods:** I have a few select favorite fast-food restaurants that are my go-to on days I just don't feel like cooking or am out running errands all day. The big difference is - I PLAN in advance. Create **designated moments** that make room to enjoy your favorite fast foods

This list does not have to be perfect. You will be updating throughout the year as you learn more about healthy food substitutions and improve your habits

KID'S TIME TO SHINE

Allow your kids to participate in putting together these meal plans! The more they are involved in meal planning and the more they learn about food, the more they will be open to trying new foods. Bonus: Start putting together a binder with all your family recipes and pictures.

FAMILY MEAL PLAN

Breakfast (*On the go!)

_____

_____

_____

_____

_____

_____

_____

_____

_____

_____

Favorite must-have fast food

_____

_____

_____

_____

Designated times fast food is OK!

_____

_____

_____

_____

Lunch/Dinner

_____

_____

_____

_____

_____

_____

_____

_____

_____

_____

_____

_____

Snacks

_____

_____

_____

_____

_____

Make a copy of this so you can stick it on your Healthy Habits board!

WEEK 11 CHALLENGE

☆ Eat a balanced breakfast every morning this week

☐ ☐ ☐ ☐ ☐ ☐ ☐

☆ Replace one of your grains with a healthier alternative that avoids the forbidden four

☐ ☐ ☐ ☐ ☐ ☐ ☐

REMEMBER, SOME HABITS HAVE TO END FOR BETTER HABITS TO BEGIN

THIS WEEK'S TOP THREE

☆ _____

☆ _____

☆ _____

Sunday

Sleep ☺ 😐 😴

Move your body

Monday

Sleep ☺ 😐 😴

Move your body

Tuesday

Sleep ☺ 😐 😴

Move your body

Wednesday

Sleep 🙂 😐 😴

Move your body

Thursday

Sleep 🙂 😐 😴

Move your body

Friday

Sleep 🙂 😐 😴

Move your body

Saturday

Sleep 🙂 😐 😴

Move your body

Something new I learned...

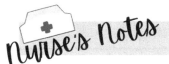

Challenge: *Eat a balanced breakfast every day this weekk*

Breakfast means to break away your fast from not eating through the night. Eating breakfast is important because it replenishes your body's energy to fuel your brain and muscles to get you ready for the day. Without breakfast, the body gets stressed and taps into its reserved energy, sometimes from the muscles. This is especially important for children because their metabolic needs are higher than adults.

- **Breakfast fuels the brain and muscles.** Research shows that kids and adults who eat breakfast perform better in school and at work

- **Breakfast improves your behavior and mood**. Stable blood sugar is critical in fueling the brain to manage emotions and make the right decisions. Tackling a day's worth of challenges is difficult when your brain and body is hungry or nutrient-deprived

- **Eating breakfast can help manage weight**. If you skip a meal, your hunger level increases and you're at risk for overeating or eating junk food. PLANNING a healthy breakfast ahead of time will set you up to make better choices throughout the day

Breakfast ideas

A perfect breakfast includes a balance of **complex carbohydrates** and **proteins**. This combination helps the brain work at its best.

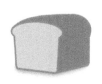

- Whole-grain English muffin with peanut butter and banana
- Whole-grain waffles topped with greek yogurt and berries
- Whole-grain toast with cheese and scrambled eggs
- Oatmeal topped with choice of nuts and fruit
- Whole-grain tortilla filled with cheese and egg

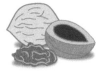

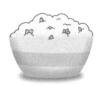

CHOOSING A PACKAGED BREAKFAST

Challenge: *Replace one of your grains with a healthier alternative that avoids the forbidden four*

Packaged breakfasts have become a staple in busy homes. It's important to choose a balanced breakfast to power you through the day. Review the lesson on the ingredients list in week 3. When choosing a packaged breakfast, try to find one that fits these criteria.

☐ Which ingredients are listed first? Ex. Look for "whole wheat". Not just wheat.
☐ At least 3 grams of protein per serving
☐ At least 3 grams of fiber per serving
☐ Less than 6 grams of sugar (more than this, I consider it "dessert")
☐ No forbidden four - high fructose corn syrup, hydrogenated oils, artificial sugars, or artificial colors

nurse's notes

HEALTHY CARBS VS JUNK CARBS

Healthy Carbs

✓ Complex carbohydrates (whole grains, legumes, vegetables, nuts)

✓ Includes proteins and fiber

✓ Absorbed more slowly in the blood, which provides steady levels of energy released over time

✓ Help you stay satisfied longer

✓ Ex. An apple has fiber, which slows the digestion of the sugars for steady release of energy

Junk carbs

✓ Simple carbohydrates

✓ Minimal to no protein or fiber

✓ Enters blood fast, quick energy released, but doesn't last long

✓ Stresses out the brain - hungry and irritable faster

✓ Ex. Apple juice does not have fiber to slow the sugar down

KID'S TIME TO SHINE

Smart shopping tip: Have your kids carry a loaf of white bread in one hand and a loaf of whole wheat bread in the other hand. Notice the white bread is much lighter, because it has no nutrients. Whole grain bread is heavier, because it is dense with nutrients

WEEK 12 CHALLENGE

☆ Plan your breakfast ahead of time every day this week

☐ ☐ ☐ ☐ ☐ ☐ ☐

☆ Review M&M Moments - Tips on introducing new foods

THERE WILL BE TOUGH TIMES, BUT OVERCOMING THOSE TIMES GIVES YOU CONTROL
YOU WILL BE PROUD!

THIS WEEK'S TOP THREE

☆ _____

☆ _____

☆ _____

⬡ Sunday

Sleep ☺ 😐 😪

Breakfast:

Move your body

⬡ Monday

Sleep ☺ 😐 😪

Breakfast:

Move your body

⬡ Tuesday

Sleep ☺ 😐 😪

Breakfast:

Move your body

Wednesday

Sleep 🙂 😐 😴 Breakfast:

Move your body

Thursday

Sleep 🙂 😐 😴 Breakfast:

Move your body

Friday

Sleep 🙂 😐 😴 Breakfast:

Move your body

Saturday

Sleep 🙂 😐 😴 Breakfast:

Move your body

I am proud of myself for...

M&M MOMENT

Challenge: *Plan your breakfast ahead of time every day this week*

One reason we resort to junk food is we did not plan ahead, or we're in a rush and don't have time to prepare anything healthy. Don't trust your hungriest self to make smart food decisions. Practice planning ahead. Writing the foods you're going to eat sets your intentions. See what works for you - planning a week in advance or planning your foods the night before.

Benefits of a Food journal

Journaling is a way of talking to yourself. Oftentimes, you will find solutions to your problems just by writing it out. For example, when you write down the foods you eat, research shows...

→ You become more aware of your eating habits - what you eat, how much you eat, how often you eat, why you eat, and when you eat
→ It helps you reach your goals by being able to analyze your habits, put them into perspective, and identify what needs to be changed
→ You cut down on mindless or emotional eating
→ You save lots of money! $$

Sample Breakfast Plan

Wednesday
Sleep 🙂 😐 😆
Move your body
Breakfast:
Whole grain cereal with.
- greek yogurt, or
- walnuts and berries

Thursday
Sleep 🙂 😐 😆
Move your body
Breakfast:
Oatmeal with.
- walnuts and berries, or
- peanut butter and banana

Friday
Sleep 🙂 😐 😆
Move your body
Breakfast:
Sweet potato with.
- egg and spinach, or
- sausage and egg

Saturday
Sleep 🙂 😐 😆
Move your body
Breakfast:
Whole grain toast with.
- scrambled egg and avocado, or
- peanut butter and banana

To increase success in meal planning, allow your family to help pick out their food for the week. Then each morning, give your family slightly different options to allow your kids some autonomy and flexibility.

Expert status: Prepare all the foods the night before, so it is easier to put together or grab and go in the morning!

Nurse's Notes — TIPS ON INTRODUCING NEW FOODS

Your taste buds regenerate every 2 weeks! Continue exposing your family to new foods, and your taste buds may begin to enjoy foods you didn't like before.

PHASES OF TRYING NEW FOODS

1. I'm only eating this because it provides nutrients to my body, I don't particularly enjoy it
2. This meal is just OK, but it's not my favorite either
3. I like this meal because it makes me feel good
4. I LOVE this meal, it's one of my favorites! I start to crave for it.

→ It takes at least 10-15 times of exposing your kids to a new food before they even try it, so don't give up!

→ Don't pressure! Trying new foods should be an enjoyable experience, if they don't like it, it's OK. They can try again later prepared a different way

→ Pair a new food with something they already like. For example, if they like eating pepperoni pizza, try adding a few mushrooms to it

→ Use the function of foods to encourage them to eat based on their interest. Ex. "These foods help you grow, these foods slow you down"

"Eating sweet potatoes has nutrients to help you grow strong muscles to climb the monkey bars at the park and it helps prevent you from getting sick."
"Eating blueberries is like food for the brain. Eat blueberries and study hard, you'll do really well on that test coming up!"

These don't happen overnight, but the more we prioritize these foods, your family WILL see a difference in health and behavior.

Check out these flashcards made especially for children to learn how certain foods can benefit their bodies! www.anti-inflammatoryliving.com/foodflashcards

→ Be a role model! Try new foods as a family and stay positive during the experience. It's OK to not like something new, but acknowledge that you are all doing a great job finding new ways to nourish your body!

MONTHLY REFLECTION

Use this time to review your vision board and update as needed!

☆ A moment I can't forget...

☆ The hardest thing about this past month was...

☆ We got through the hardest times together by...

☆ I am so proud of...

☆ Best meal I thouroughly enjoyed:

☆ We're one step closer to our goals because...

KID'S TIME TO SHINE

Space for your kids to write or draw what they enjoyed the most this last month

MONTHLY HABIT TRACKER

Print one out for each family member & post it on your family board! Track the habits you are concentrating on. Color it in after completing it and celebrate every day's win! 1 symbol = 1 day.

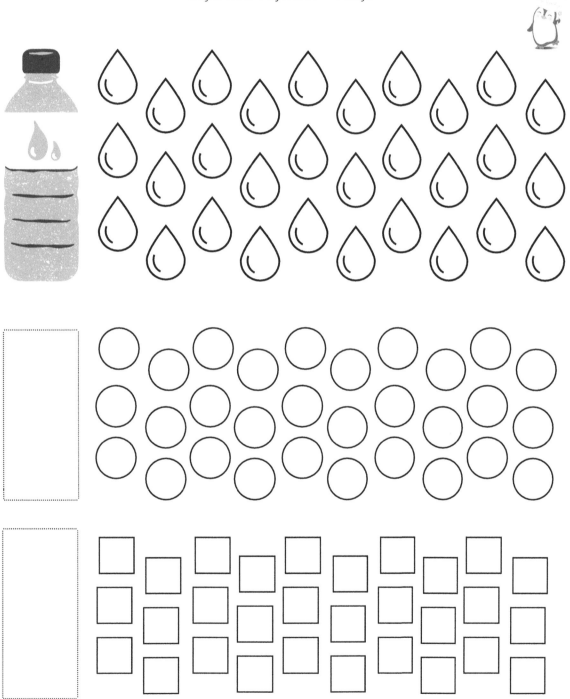

WEEK 13 CHALLENGE

☆ Review nurse's notes - Why is protein so important?

☐ ☐ ☐ ☐ ☐ ☐ ☐

☆ Make a list of your favorite protein snacks

You don't have to eat less,
you have to eat right

THIS WEEK'S TOP THREE

☆ _____

☆ _____

☆ _____

Sunday

Sleep 🙂 😐 😫

Move your body

Breakfast:

Monday

Sleep 🙂 😐 😫

Move your body

Breakfast:

Tuesday

Sleep 🙂 😐 😫

Move your body

Breakfast:

Wednesday

Sleep 😊 😐 😣   Breakfast:

Move your body

Thursday

Sleep 😊 😐 😣   Breakfast:

Move your body

Friday

Sleep 😊 😐 😣   Breakfast:

Move your body

Saturday

Sleep 😊 😐 😣   Breakfast:

Move your body

Something that brought me joy this week...

nurse's notes

Prioritize protein! Children need adequate protein every day to grow

- Builds and repairs bones, muscles, and all tissues. Your muscles, organs, immune system, and more all require protein for proper growth and development

- Stabilizes our blood sugar. Eating protein slows the absorption of sugars and carbohydrates, which also help keep you full longer

- Boosts immune system. Adequate protein provides the building blocks for your immune system to protect your body and fight infections

- Improves energy, behavior, and mood. Eating protein raises the hormones that act as a natural anti-depressant and are responsible for positive energy

Protein requirements

	CHILDREN	ADULTS
NEEDS	1 gram of protein per pound	1/2 gram of protein per 1 lb of weight
EXAMPLE	50lb child needs 50g protein	150lb adult needs 75g protein

*Children need more protein per lb of weight because their little bodies use up more energy than adults, and need it to grow

great protein options

2 tablespoons of peanut butter = 8 g of protein

1 cup of oatmeal = 6 g of protein

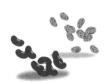

1 egg = 6 g of protein

1 cup milk = 8 g of protein

1 serving greek yogurt = 15 g of protein

4 oz chicken breast = 25 g of protein

100 g of beans = 9 gm of protein

PROTEIN SNACKS

Challenge: *Make a list of your favorite protein snacks, bonus points for quick store-bought snacks!*

Sometimes, we need a quick snack to keep us going through the day, or in between meals. This is important to have ESPECIALLY when traveling with kids! I empower you to primarily carry healthy snacks as opposed to junk food in your home. Find your favorite high-protein snacks and always have that with you wherever you go

Protein snacks

_____

_____

_____

_____

_____

_____

_____

_____

_____

_____

Mine and my kid's favorite quick protein snacks I always have when on the go...

- string cheese

- bag of nuts

- hard boiled egg

(no affiliation, my kids just love these!)

- beef or chicken jerky sticks (Snack Mates)

- Cerebelly granola bars

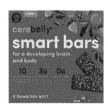 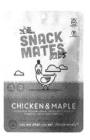

KID'S TIME TO SHINE

I usually have these as "anytime snacks" that are available for my children to snack on throughout the day or while on the go. Help your kids learn to pick a handful of snacks that meet your criteria and give your children the choice of which to eat to allow them some autonomy and flexibility.

WEEK 14 CHALLENGE

☆ Add at least TWO servings of fruits each day

☐ ☐ ☐ ☐ ☐ ☐ ☐

☆ Review nurse's notes: Why are fruits so important?

☆ Kid's Time to Shine Activity

Eating well is a form of *self-love and respect*

THIS WEEK'S TOP THREE

☆ _____

☆ _____

☆ _____

Sunday

Sleep 😊 😐 😫

Move your body

Breakfast:

Monday

Sleep 😊 😐 😫

Move your body

Breakfast:

Tuesday

Sleep 😊 😐 😫

Move your body

Breakfast:

Wednesday

Sleep 🙂 😐 😣   Breakfast:

Move your body

Thursday

Sleep 🙂 😐 😣   Breakfast:

Move your body

Friday

Sleep 🙂 😐 😣   Breakfast:

Move your body

Saturday

Sleep 🙂 😐 😣   Breakfast:

Move your body

Share a favorite memory that always make you smile...

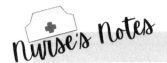

FRUITS AND VEGETABLES

Challenge: *Add at least TWO servings of fruits per day*

Why is it so important?

CDC research study says that American children and adults are not eating adequate fruits and vegetables.

- Only 1 in 10 adults eat their fruits and vegetable recommendations [1]
- Only 7.1% of adolescents age 14-18 eat their recommended fruit intake [2]
- Only 2% of adolescents age 14-18 eat their recommended vegetable intake [2]

These research findings are terrible! A few reasons why the adequate intake of fruits and vegetables is essential to our daily living...

- Low in calories
- High in vitamins, minerals
- High in fiber
- High in phytochemicals
- Heals our brains and bodies
- Reduces and protects against inflammation

Over the next few weeks, you'll learn what this actually means to our growing children and as adults. But in the meantime, let's work on ways we can include it in our diets knowing that it reduces the risk of diet-related chronic disease

- Heart disease
- Diabetes
- Obesity
- Some cancers

... and so much more!

KID'S TIME TO SHINE

Shop the colors of the rainbow. This is a great way to introduce new fruits and vegetables to your kids. In the produce section of the store, have each of your kids pick out at least 3 different colors of fruits and vegetables to try at home.

1 Only 1 in 10 Adults Get Enough Fruits or Vegetables. CDC. 2017. https://www.cdc.gov/media/releases/2017/p1116-fruit-vegetable-consumption.html.

2 Percentage of Adolescents Meeting Federal Fruit and Vegetable Intake Recommendations - Youth Risk Behavior Surveillance System, United States, 2017. CDC. 2021. https://www.cdc.gov/mmwr/volumes/70/wr/mm7003a1.htm.

EAT THE RAINBOW

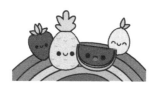

It is important to eat a variety of fruits and vegetables because the different colors provide different benefits to your body

Red

Ex. Strawberries, cranberries, tomatoes, red onions, beets, watermelon, cherries
- Protects the heart by reducing high blood pressure, high cholesterol, and atherosclerosis
- Reduces risk of cancer, diabetes, improves brain function, skin health and more

Blue and purple

Ex. Blueberries, grapes, eggplants, plums, purple potatoes, purple cabbage
- Promotes healthy digestion and urinary tract health
- Promotes healthy aging and memory function by fighting inflammation
- Reduces risk of heart disease, stroke, and cancer

Green
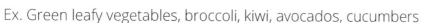

Ex. Green leafy vegetables, broccoli, kiwi, avocados, cucumbers
- Protects eyes, promotes healthy digestion, and improves immune system
- Reduces risk of cancer and helps detoxify the body
- Promotes strong bones and teeth, healthy heart and blood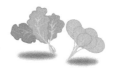
- One of the healthiest foods to eat, highest in antioxidants and fiber

yellow and orange
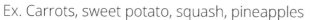

Ex. Carrots, sweet potato, squash, pineapples
- Protects brain health, eye health, and prevent heart disease and stroke
- Maintain skin health, improves immune system, build strong teeth and bones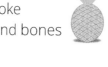

White

Ex. Bananas, onions, mushrooms, cauliflower, garlic
- Protects heart by reducing high blood pressure and high cholesterol
- Improves immune system and reduces risk of cancer

WEEK 15 CHALLENGE

☆ Add at least TWO servings of fruits each day

☐ ☐ ☐ ☐ ☐ ☐ ☐

☆ Add at least TWO servings vegetables each day

☐ ☐ ☐ ☐ ☐ ☐ ☐

☆ Review nurse's notes: Fiber

YOUR DIET IS A BANK ACCOUNT, YOUR FOOD CHOICES ARE YOUR INVESTMENT

- BETHANY FRANKEL

THIS WEEK'S TOP THREE

☆ _____

☆ _____

☆ _____

Sunday

Sleep ☺ 😐 😴

Move your body

Breakfast:

Monday

Sleep ☺ 😐 😴

Move your body

Breakfast:

Tuesday

Sleep ☺ 😐 😴

Move your body

Breakfast:

Wednesday

Sleep 😊 😐 😴   Breakfast:

Move your body

Thursday

Sleep 😊 😐 😴   Breakfast:

Move your body

Friday

Sleep 😊 😐 😴   Breakfast:

Move your body

Saturday

Sleep 😊 😐 😴   Breakfast:

Move your body

I am thankful for...

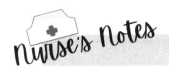

FRUITS AND VEGETABLES

Challenge: *Add at least TWO servings of fruits per day and add at least TWO servings of vegetables per day*

────────────────── *Tips* ──────────────────

✓ Try to fit in as many food groups in each meal - Fresh veggies or salad before the main dish and a side of fruit after. This is where you get really good at portion control to try to fit all these foods in one meal!

✓ Eat an apple first thing in the morning. Did you know - an apple has enough nutrients to kick start your day as much as a cup of coffee will do? Without the caffeine fix of course

✓ **It takes at least 10-15 times of exposing your kids to new foods before they may even try it, so don't give up! Review week 11 tips**

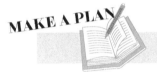

PROMISE TO MYSELF

Write down ideas on what and when you will eat these fruits and veggies

Favorite fruits & veggies

ex. strawberry or sliced apple and spinach salad before dinner

_____

_____

_____

_____

_____

_____

_____

New fruits & veggies to try

ex. add chopped asparagus to dinner casseroles

_____

_____

_____

_____

_____

_____

_____

WHAT'S SO SPECIAL ABOUT FIBER?

Fiber Improves the health of your gut bacteria, which can increase your happy hormones, decrease risks of heart disease, diabetes, diverticular disease, constipation, and some cancers. There are 2 main categories of fiber...

Soluble Fiber

ex. Oatmeal, nuts, beans, apples, blueberries

- Helps lower blood sugar

- Helps lower blood cholesterol

Insoluble Fiber

ex.Whole wheat bread, brown rice, carrots, cucumbers, tomatoes.

- Helps move food through the digestive system, prevents constipation

Daily Fiber Requirements

	CHILDREN	ADULTS
NEEDS	ADD 5 grams to their age	At least 25 g a day
EXAMPLE	5 year old needs 10 g of fiber	-

Increase Fiber Intake

- **Eat whole fruits and vegetables** instead of drinking juice. The peels in apples contain fiber that isn't found in apple juice

- **Eat whole-grain** instead of white. Look for the word "WHOLE" in ingredients, not just wheat when choosing bread or cereals

- **Love beans**. Almost all types of beans and peas are rich sources of fiber. Throw it in your salad, soups, casseroles, or on the side of any dish

- Find a **high fiber cereal**. At least 3 grams per serving

- **Sprinkle seeds on every meal**: Flaxseed, chia seed, pumpkin seeds, etc

WEEK 16 CHALLENGE

☆ Add at least THREE servings
of vegetables each day

☐ ☐ ☐ ☐ ☐ ☐ ☐

☆ Are you still drinking enough
water?

☐ ☐ ☐ ☐ ☐ ☐ ☐

It doesn't matter
how slow you go,
as long as you
don't give up

THIS WEEK'S TOP THREE

☆ _____

☆ _____

☆ _____

Sunday

Sleep 😊 😐 😴

Move your body

Breakfast:

Monday

Sleep 😊 😐 😴

Move your body

Breakfast:

Tuesday

Sleep 😊 😐 😴

Move your body

Breakfast:

Wednesday

Sleep 🙂 😐 😫   Breakfast:

Move your body

Thursday

Sleep 🙂 😐 😫   Breakfast:

Move your body

Friday

Sleep 🙂 😐 😫   Breakfast:

Move your body

Saturday

Sleep 🙂 😐 😫   Breakfast:

Move your body

Something I handled well...

MORE VEGETABLES PLEASE

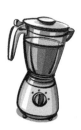

We love blended smoothies! Sometimes, I make it extra thick and creamy, and my kids call it ice cream. #winning. Blended smoothies are a super easy way to get ALL your servings of fruits, vegetables, and more nutrients in one "meal." Or it can be split up and sipped on throughout the day! I freeze leftovers into popsicles.

Smoothie Tips

You can find several recipes by searching Google or Pinterest. So instead of sharing recipes, I will share my best tips.

- **Use frozen fruits and vegetables.** They last longer, less waste, and save money! It's easier since cutting or prepping is not needed. Measure, throw in a blender, and get that thick, ice cream-like consistency!

- Frozen chopped **kale** and frozen chopped **spinach** are the best vegetables to start with because of their mild flavor

- Adding **bananas** (for smooth creamy flavors) or **pineapples** (for citrus flavors) are the best fruits to add as a base because they can mask the flavors of vegetables

- Add frozen **cauliflower!** It doesn't add any flavor, no one will know it's there, but it creates the same creaminess as bananas and is a superfood

- Add a **handful of walnuts** for healthy fats and protein to slow down the burst of sugars from all the fruits. Walnuts are also a mild flavor and can be masked easily by the fruits

- Add **chia seeds** or **flax seeds** for additional healthy fats, proteins, and fiber. These super seeds have little to no flavor and are dense in nutrients

FB POST

What's in your blender? Post in our FB community!

MORE VEGETABLES PLEASE

More fun and creative ways to include vegetables in your meals

- **DIP.** Dip sliced raw or roasted vegetables in hummus, guacamole, cream cheese, tomato sauce, or your favorite salad dressing

- **TOP.** Roast or steam vegetables, then top it with your favorite toppings, such as melted cheese, uncured bacon bits, roasted garlic, etc

- **SNEAK.** Add grated or thinly sliced vegetables to your favorite meals... Grated cauliflower has a mild flavor and is easily masked in macaroni and cheese. Chopped spinach also picks up the flavor of most cooked dishes, great in spaghetti or fried rice

- **SIP.** Blend vegetables into your favorite soups

- **FILL.** Stuff vegetables in either a whole wheat tortilla for quesadilla style, in whole wheat bread for grilled cheese style, or with eggs in an omelet. Bonus: Then DIP IT in hummus, tomato sauce, or guacamole!

KID'S TIME TO SHINE

These are great ways to get your kids involved. Let them play with their food! Kids learn best through exploration and play. They may be willing to try new foods if they play with them first by being involved in the preparation.

- **PIZZA.** Make your own pizza day. Prepare a handful of ingredients, including vegetables, of course, and encourage your family to put at least 2 or 3 types of vegetables on their pizza

- **DESIGN.** Arrange food into a face, a boat, or shape your children desires

- **GROW.** Start a small garden, so they can appreciate the process of growing their own fruits and vegetables

MONTHLY REFLECTION

Use this time to review your vision board and update as needed!

☆ What were your family's biggest accomplishments?

☆ What were your biggest fears/stressors?

☆ How did you or do you plan on overcoming those fears/stressors?

☆ Have you noticed any changes in your family, such as behavior, symptoms or etc.?

☆ I am so proud of...

☆ Best meal I thouroughly enjoyed:

KID'S TIME TO SHINE

 Space for your kids to write or draw what they enjoyed the most this last month

MONTHLY HABIT TRACKER

Print one out for each family member & post it on your family board! Track the habits you are concentrating on. Color it in after completing it and celebrate every day's win! 1 symbol = 1 day.

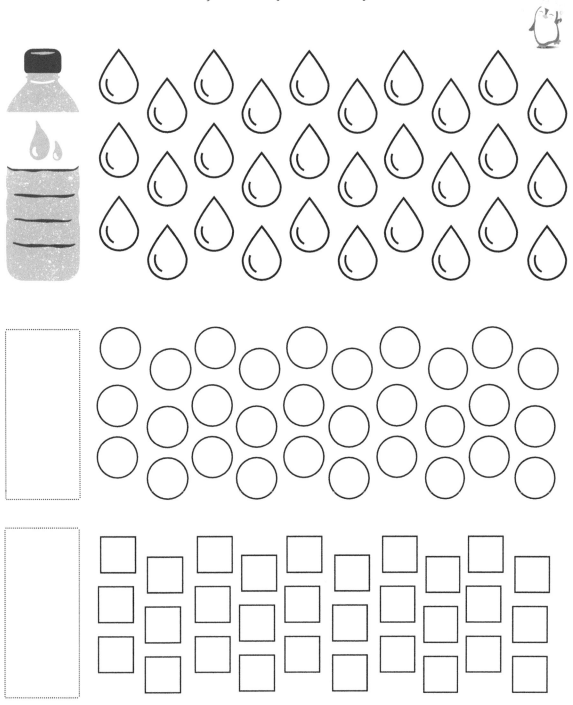

☆ Pick one new habit from previous weeks you still need work on

☐ ☐ ☐ ☐ ☐ ☐ ☐

☆ Send a message to someone each day to express your gratitude.

☐ ☐ ☐ ☐ ☐ ☐ ☐

It is not joy that makes us grateful, it is *Gratitude* that makes us joyful

THIS WEEK'S TOP THREE

☆ _____

☆ _____
_____

☆ _____

Sunday

Sleep 😊 😐 😣

Move your body

Breakfast:

Monday

Sleep 😊 😐 😣

Move your body

Breakfast:

Tuesday

Sleep 😊 😐 😣

Move your body

Breakfast:

Wednesday

Sleep 🙂 😐 😴   Breakfast:

Move your body

Thursday

Sleep 🙂 😐 😴   Breakfast:

Move your body

Friday

Sleep 🙂 😐 😴   Breakfast:

Move your body

Saturday

Sleep 🙂 😐 😴   Breakfast:

Move your body

A person I appreciated...

☆ Avoid fast food this week!

☐ ☐ ☐ ☐ ☐ ☐ ☐

☆ Review Nurse's Notes

☆ Find and write a positive
affirmation on a post-it, post it
on every mirror you have in
your home

THE FOOD YOU EAT
CAN EITHER BE THE
MOST POWERFUL FORM
OF MEDICINE, OR THE
SLOWEST FORM OF
POISON

THIS WEEK'S TOP THREE

☆ _____

☆ _____

☆ _____

Sunday

Sleep ☺ 😐 😴

Breakfast:

Move your body

Monday

Sleep ☺ 😐 😠

Breakfast:

Move your body

Tuesday

Sleep ☺ 😐 😠

Breakfast:

Move your body

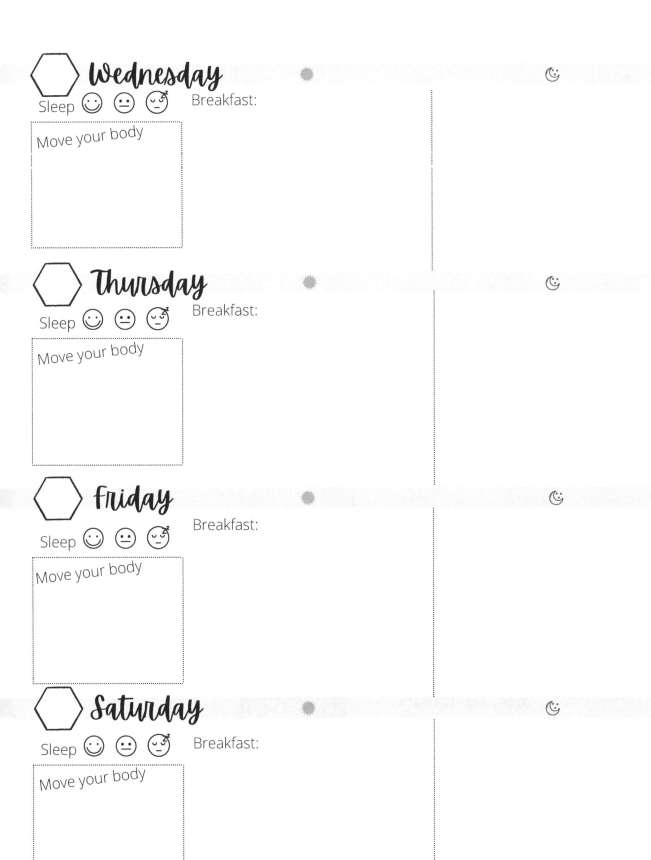

Wednesday

Sleep 🙂 😐 😴   Breakfast:

Move your body

Thursday

Sleep 🙂 😐 😴   Breakfast:

Move your body

Friday

Sleep 🙂 😐 😴   Breakfast:

Move your body

Saturday

Sleep 🙂 😐 😴   Breakfast:

Move your body

Something new I learned...

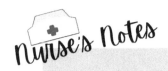

DANGERS OF HIGH SALT

Challenge: *Avoid fast food this week!*

Salt is made of sodium and chloride. Your body does need some sodium to maintain a balance between water and minerals, contract and relax muscles, and conduct nerve impulses. But salt is found in so many foods nowadays, it's easy to consume too much. Too much salt could disrupt those processes and cause high blood pressure, heart disease, and stroke.

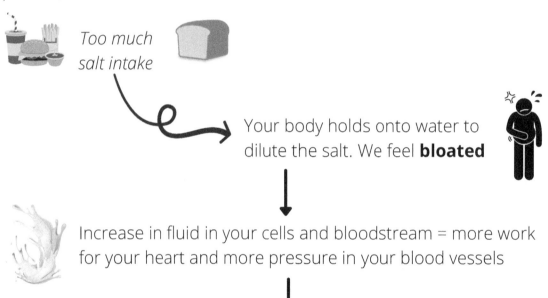

Too much salt intake

Your body holds onto water to dilute the salt. We feel **bloated**

↓

Increase in fluid in your cells and bloodstream = more work for your heart and more pressure in your blood vessels

↓

More pressure on your blood vessels makes them stiff overtime = **arteriosclerosis**

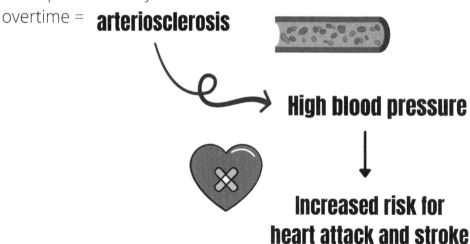

High blood pressure

↓

Increased risk for heart attack and stroke

TOP 10 SOURCES OF SODIUM

1. Bread

2. Pizza

3. Sandwiches

4. Cold cuts, Cured meats, canned meats

5. Soups

6. Burritos, Tacos

7. Savory Snacks (chips, popcorn, pretzels, crackers)

8. Chicken

9. Cheese

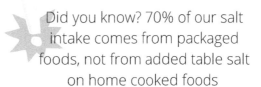

Did you know? 70% of our salt intake comes from packaged foods, not from added table salt on home cooked foods

10. Eggs, Omelets

MAKE A PLAN

How often do you eat any of these foods? Avoid fast food this week, but make a plan to decrease your salt intake moving forward.

Promise to myself: _____

_____

_____

_____

_____

Top 10 Sources of Sodium. 2021. CDC. https://www.cdc.gov/salt/sources.htm

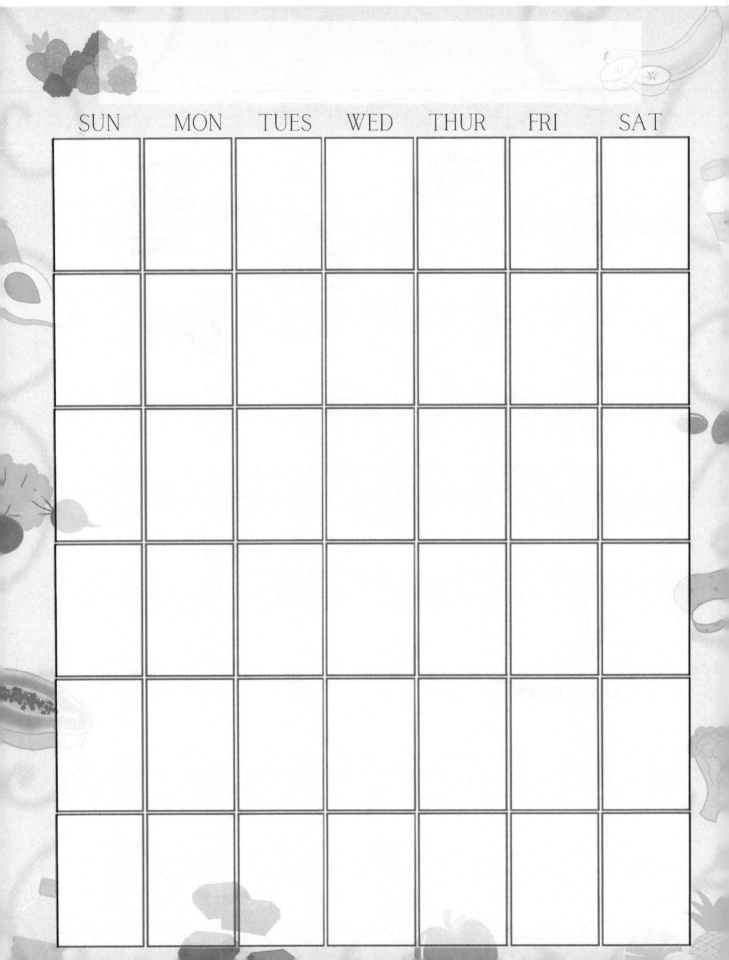

SUN	MON	TUES	WED	THUR	FRI	SAT

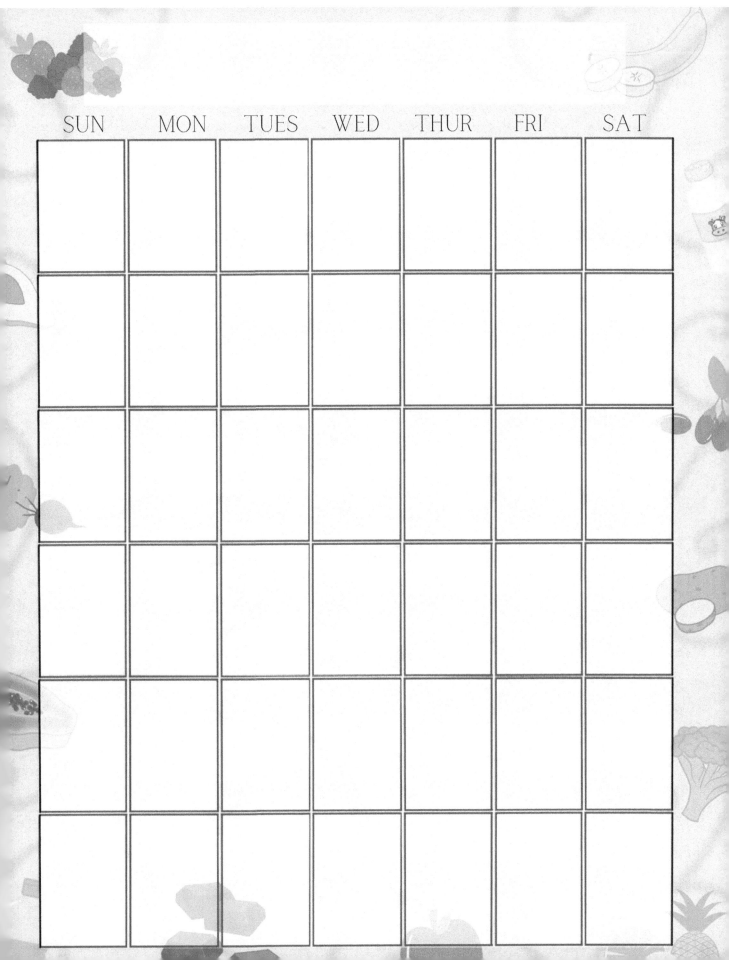

SUN	MON	TUES	WED	THUR	FRI	SAT

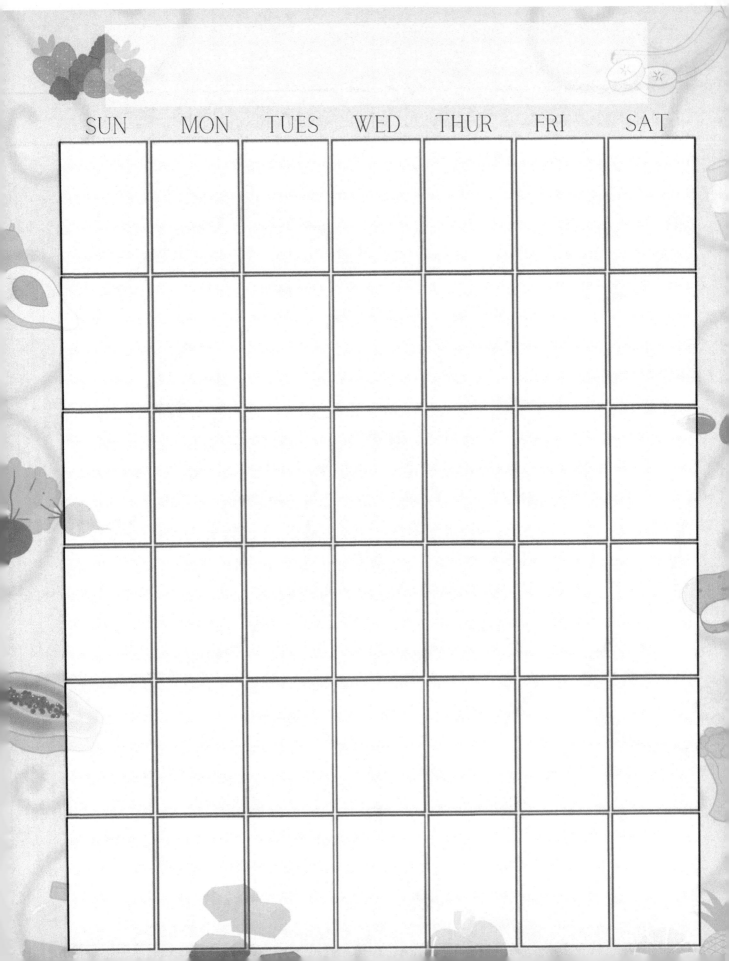

SUN	MON	TUES	WED	THUR	FRI	SAT

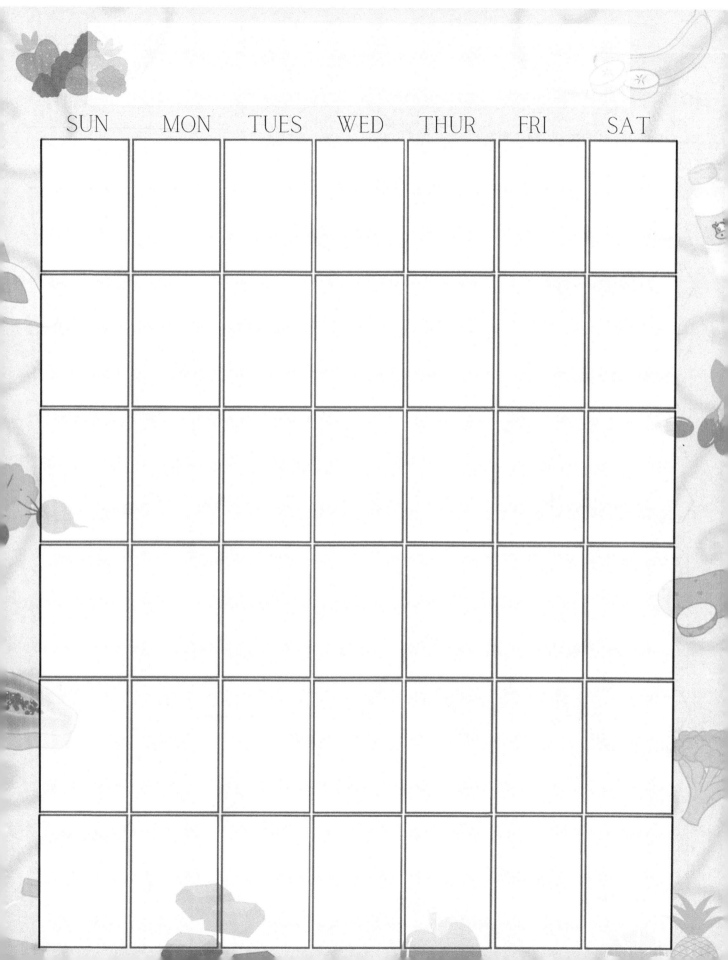

SUN	MON	TUES	WED	THUR	FRI	SAT

☆ Ingredient's check! What's in your cooking oil, butter, cheese? Replace at least one of these with a healthier alternative.

☆ Add a serving of Omega 3's to at least one meal a day.

☐ ☐ ☐ ☐ ☐ ☐ ☐

I CAN'T CONTROL EVERYTHING IN LIFE. BUT I CAN CONTROL WHAT I PUT IN MY BODY

THIS WEEK'S TOP THREE

☆ _____

☆ _____

☆ _____

Sunday

Sleep 😊 😐 😴

Breakfast:

Move your body

Monday

Sleep 😊 😐 😴

Breakfast:

Move your body

Tuesday

Sleep 😊 😐 😴

Breakfast:

Move your body

Wednesday

Sleep 🙂 😐 😩 Breakfast:

Move your body

Thursday

Sleep 🙂 😐 😩 Breakfast:

Move your body

Friday

Sleep 🙂 😐 😩 Breakfast:

Move your body

Saturday

Sleep 🙂 😐 😩 Breakfast:

Move your body

I am proud of myself for...

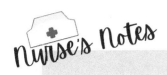
nurse's Notes

THE FACTS ABOUT FAT

Fats are a part of every cell in your body. We need it to survive. Your hormones and metabolism need fat, your brain nerve cells are made of fat, in fact, fat makes up 60% of your brain!

The benefits of eating the right fats include...

- Required to absorb vitamins A, D, E, and K

- Maintain healthy hair and skin

- Provides energy

- Helps foods taste great and helps you feel full

Did you know?
One of the most potent foods containing healthy fats is BREAST MILK! Studies show the longer an infant breastfeeds, the risks of many mental and physical diseases decrease

The brains of young children grow rapidly in the first five years. They need adequate amounts of fat to help their brains develop normally and optimally. Feeding them healthy fats can help build a foundation for future success in learning and health.

— *Example* —

Challenge: *Ingredient's check! What's in your cooking oil, butter, cheese? Replace at least one of these with a healthier alternative.*

Review Week 3's Ingredient's Label for a refresher... Choose your foods wisely!

☐ Choose foods with monounsaturated fats or polyunsaturated fats

☐ Eat less saturated fats

☐ Avoid trans fat

☐ Avoid the "forbidden four"

Remember this...
Even if the package says ZERO TRANS FAT, the food can legally contain half a gram of trans fat. That's why checking the ingredients label is most important and reliable!

Ingredients from a popular block of cheese for melting

Milk, whey, skim milk, milk protein concentrate, water, milkfat, whey protein concentrate, sodium phosphate, modified food starch, contains less than 2% of salt, calcium phosphate, dried corn syrup, canola oil, maltodextrin, lactic acid, sorbic acid as preservative, sodium alginate, sodium citrate, cheese culture, enzymes, apocarotenal, and annatto (color).

Ingredients from a block of REAL cheese

Cultured pasteurized organic milk, salt, microbial enzymes

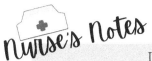

IT'S TIME FOR AN OIL CHANGE!

Challenge: *Add a serving of Omega 3's to at least one meal a day*

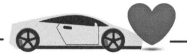

Your body is like a car. Your heart is like the engine. You know how important it is to maintain your car by getting regular oil changes and filling up your tank with the right kind of fuel, or gas. If you use the wrong oil or the wrong kind of gas, it can mess up your engine and decrease the life of the car. Your heart is the same. Over time, using the wrong kinds of oil and fuel, or food, will overwhelm your body and decrease your quality of life due to the increased risk of chronic medical conditions.

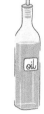

→ Best oils I use? Olive oil for light cooking, avocado oil for higher heat cooking

Benefits of Omega 3's

Omega 3's (EPA and DHA) are one of the healthiest nutrients we can take that is found in fats or as a supplement

- Builds healthy brain cells
- Improves mood, decreases depression
- Improves learning and attention span
- Protects against Alzheimer's and dementia

- Decreases pain and inflammation
- Improves eczema
- Lowers cholesterol
- Decreases risk of some cancers

and so much more!!

Omega 3's are potent in the following foods...
- Salmon, sardines, and other fishes
- Walnuts, flax seeds, chia seeds
- Organic, grass-fed beef and omega 3 enriched eggs

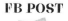

FB POST What ingredient are you replacing and what new healthier alternative did you find? Check out our Facebook community for some ideas!

☆ Pantry Scavenger Hunt:
Sugar High

☆ Replace one of your food
items with one without
added sugar

HEALTH IS A
DAILY PRACTICE.
NOT A 30-DAY DIET

☆ _____

☆ _____

☆ _____

Sunday

Sleep 😊 😐 😣

Move your body

Breakfast:

Monday

Sleep 😊 😐 😣

Move your body

Breakfast:

Tuesday

Sleep 😊 😐 😣

Move your body

Breakfast:

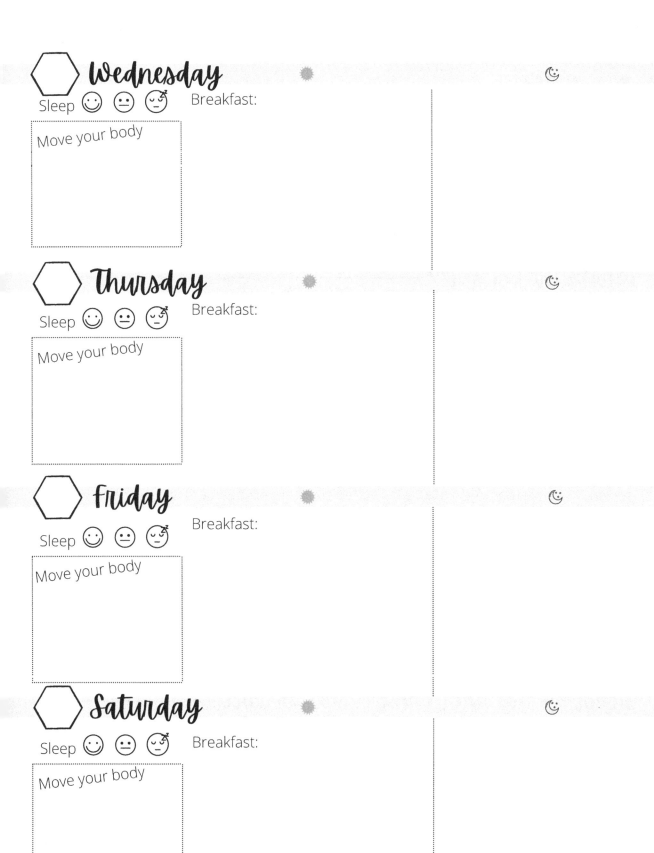

Wednesday

Sleep ☺ 😐 😣

Breakfast:

Move your body

Thursday

Sleep ☺ 😐 😣

Breakfast:

Move your body

Friday

Sleep ☺ 😐 😣

Breakfast:

Move your body

Saturday

Sleep ☺ 😐 😣

Breakfast:

Move your body

Something that brought me joy this week...

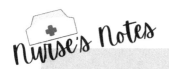

SUGAR HIGH

Did you know?

Sugar is found in SO MANY foods. Check for ADDED sugars in your bread, tortilla, ketchup, bacon, spaghetti sauce, peanut butter, yogurts, salad dressings, canned fruits, non-dairy milks, and more!

What's the big deal?

Excessive intake of sugar can increase your risk of obesity, metabolic syndrome, type 2 diabetes, and more. This does not happen because of the occasional birthday cake or ice cream you treat yourself with, it's because many people are unaware of how much sugar is in the foods they eat every day!

How much sugar is recommended?

Added sugar for children and adults should stay under 10% of total calories. Don't be fooled by a label that says "only 1g" of added sugar. 1g of sugar adds up over time! If you can find an alternative to avoid it, do so. *Infants 2 and under should not eat or drink anything with added sugar at all

	CHILDREN (ages 3+)*	ADULTS
MAX	25g - 45g	50 g of sugar per day

WHO calls on countries to reduce sugars intake among adults and children. 2015. World Health Organization. https://www.who.int/news/item/04-03-2015-who-calls-on-countries-to-reduce-sugars-intake-among-adults-and-children.

Sugar by any other name is still as sweet

SUGAR

Malt sugar   Sucrose   Honey   High fructose corn syrup

Fruit juice concentrates   Agave   Dextrin   Brown sugar

Maple syrup   Corn syrup   Dextrose   Rice syrup   Maltose

Molasses   Crystalline Fructose   Maltodextrin   and more!

*Natural sweeteners such as maple syrup, honey and coconut sugar have added health benefits! Choose these over refined sugar

PANTRY SCAVENGER HUNT: SUGAR HIGH

Challenge: *Replace one of your food items with one without added sugar*

Use the **3-6-3 rule**. Any more sugar is considered dessert to me! Use this checklist when purchasing new foods.

☐ Under 6g of total sugars, ideally no "added sugars"
☐ At least 3g of protein and at least 3g of fiber
☐ Identify the types of sugars in the ingredients - is it from natural sources or not?
☐ Avoid the "forbidden four"

Total sugars vs added sugars

This is my kid's favorite granola bar. (No affiliation, we just love these!) Notice how there are still 6g of sugar, but NO ADDED sugars. This means it contains **naturally occurring** sugars in the ingredients, such as from fruit or milk. The best ones are accompanied by adequate protein and fiber. This is necessary to slow down the absorption of sugar, so your blood sugar doesn't spike and keeps you full much longer. Unlike 100% juice, there are no added sugars, but also has no protein or fiber to slow down the sugar rush in our body!

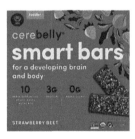

Cerebelly Smart Bars

Nutrition Facts

Servings per container (Children 1-3 years)

Serving size	1 bar (24g)

Amount per serving

Calories	90

	% Daily Value*
Total Fat 3.5g	9%
Saturated Fat 0g	0%
Trans Fat 0g	
Cholesterol 0mg	0%
Sodium 20mg	1%
Total Carbohydrate 14g	9%
Dietary Fiber 3g	21%
Total Sugars 6g	
Includes 0g Added Sugars	0%
Protein 3g	

FB POST Check our FB community for more ideas on healthier alternatives! Post what food you were most suprised about and/or a new food you're excited to try without sugar!

MONTHLY REFLECTION

Use this time to review your vision board and update as needed!

☆ A moment I can't forget...

☆ The hardest thing about this past month was...

☆ We got through the hardest times together by...

☆ I am so proud of...

☆ Best meal I thouroughly enjoyed:

☆ The funniest thing that happened was...

KID'S TIME TO SHINE

Space for your kids to write or draw what they enjoyed the most this last month

MONTHLY HABIT TRACKER

Print one out for each family member & post it on your family board! Track the habits you are concentrating on. Color it in after completing it and celebrate every day's win! 1 symbol = 1 day.

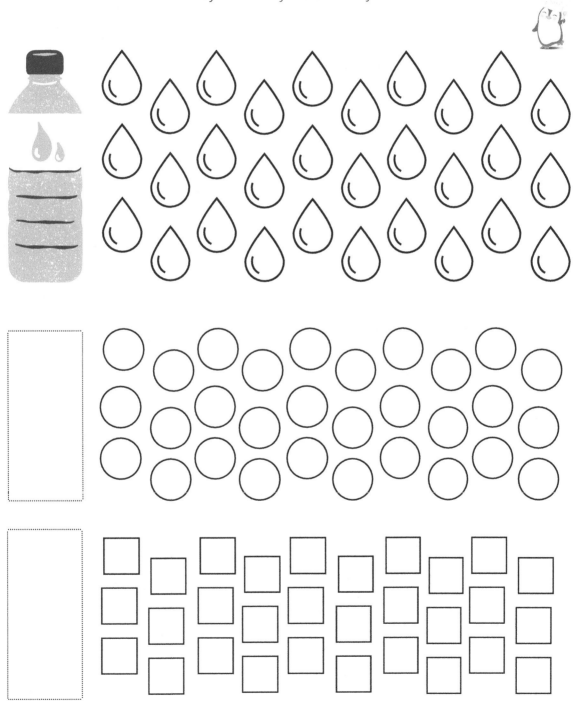

WEEK 21 CHALLENGE

☆ Put it all together - eat 3 servings of vegetables and 2 servings of fruits per day!

☐ ☐ ☐ ☐ ☐ ☐ ☐

☆ Kid's time to shine activity

A healthy outside starts from the inside

Sunday

Sleep 🙂 😐 😴

Breakfast:

Move your body

Monday

Sleep 🙂 😐 😴

Breakfast:

Move your body

Tuesday

Sleep 🙂 😐 😴

Breakfast:

Move your body

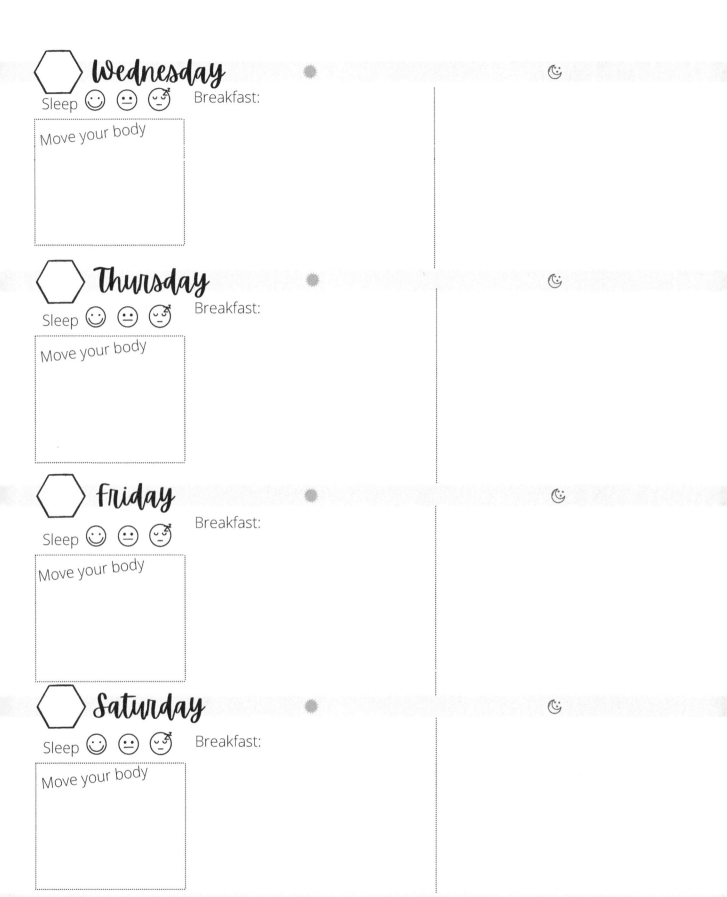

Wednesday

Sleep 🙂 😐 😴   Breakfast:

Move your body

Thursday

Sleep 🙂 😐 😴   Breakfast:

Move your body

Friday

Sleep 🙂 😐 😴   Breakfast:

Move your body

Saturday

Sleep 🙂 😐 😴   Breakfast:

Move your body

A favorite memory that always makes me smile...

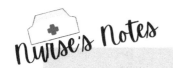

FIGHT AGAINST NATURE

What are free radicals?

Free radicals are unstable molecules. They are created when you're exposed to pollution, tobacco smoke, and UV rays. It is also a part of the normal metabolic process when you eat and digest food.

What's the big deal?

Excess free radicals in your bodies can create oxidative stress. Oxidative stress is damaging to your body.

- ✗ Increases inflammation ~> risk of autoimmune diseases and joint pains
- ✗ Damages nerve cells in the brain ~> risk of Alzheimer's and dementia
- ✗ Accelerates the aging process ~> ex. vision problems, wrinkles, hair loss
- ✗ Increased risk of heart diseases, obesity, and diabetes
- ✗ Increased risk of cancers

So, what do we do?

First, slow down on eating sugars and saturated fat, these foods cause a lot of oxidative stress. Second, enlist your personal army to combat these free radicals in your bodies! Introducing, ANTIOXIDANTS. Antioxidants are exactly what it sounds like, they are nutrients that bind to the free radicals to neutralize and prevent oxidation, therefore, preventing the risks of diseases above.

Where can I find antioxidants?

You guessed it, the most powerful antioxidants are known as phytonutrients, which are most abundant in **FRUITS AND VEGETABLES!** Other foods high in antioxidants include teas, whole grains, nuts, seeds, herbs and spices, and at least 70% cacao.

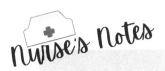

ANTIOXIDANTS

Challenge: *Add at least 2 servings of fruits and 3 servings of vegetables per day*

I know, I know. Another challenge to increase your fruits and vegetable intake! You learned a lot these last few weeks. I wanted to wrap it up by expressing how important it is again to work on this. My family's rule of thumb is: eat whatever you want, as long as you're eating enough **fruits, vegetables, and Omega 3's.**

These powerful foods have the ability to combat anything, even the harmful effects of the "worst" diets, because of their antioxidant and anti-inflammatory properties. ***When you prioritize the foods that help heal and protect your body, you can better enjoy the fun foods!***

KID'S TIME TO SHINE

See the process of oxidation and aging for yourself!

- In the morning, cut an apple and/or guacamole in half

- Squeeze lemon juice on ONE side, and leave the other side as is

Lemon juice is filled with antioxidants, vitamin C. As apples and avocados age, they turn brown. By the end of the day, notice how lemon juice prevented browning, or aging, while the other side turned brown.

....

Create a fun snack tray! This can be prepared in advance and put out in between meals. Use a charcuterie board or a muffin tin and line it up with chopped fruits and vegetables, mini sandwiches, nuts, and more. Don't forget to add an omega-3 hard-boiled egg or sprinkle chia seeds over everything for added healthy fats! Mix in "fun" foods, like their favorite candies or cookies. Even if the fun foods are eaten first, exposing them to fruits and vegetables often will work eventually!

Check out my family's favorite clean chocolate! It's made with all-natural ingredients and 70% cacao! (No affiliation). HU Chocolate - Hazelnut butter flavor :)

☆ Try something new! Include at least two top foods in your meal plan that is high in probiotics. Eat one serving a day.

☐ ☐ ☐ ☐ ☐ ☐ ☐

Happiness is a
direction
not a place

THIS WEEK'S TOP THREE

☆ _____

☆ _____

☆ _____

Sunday

Sleep ☺ ☺ ☺

Breakfast:

Move your body

Monday

Sleep ☺ ☺ ☺

Breakfast:

Move your body

Tuesday

Sleep ☺ ☺ ☺

Breakfast:

Move your body

Wednesday

◯ Sleep 🙂 😐 😫 Breakfast:

Move your body

Thursday

◯ Sleep 🙂 😐 😫 Breakfast:

Move your body

Friday

◯ Sleep 🙂 😐 😫 Breakfast:

Move your body

Saturday

◯ Sleep 🙂 😐 😫 Breakfast:

Move your body

I am thankful for...

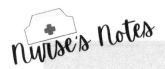

THE GOOD BACTERIA

—What is it?—

Introducing: the gut microbiome. The gut lines the digestive system, which starts from the mouth down to the rectum. The microbiome is the trillions of bacteria that live throughout the gut lining. Everyone's microbiome is as unique as your fingerprint. It is established as early as the time you spent inside your mom's womb. It is created based on what she ate while pregnant, how you were delivered, and whether you were breastfed or formula-fed. Then when you're born, it is based on your medication and antibiotic use, exposure to environmental factors such as stress and nature, lifestyle habits such as exercise and what you eat, and finally, your genetics.

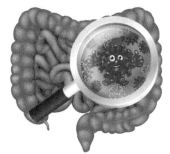

—What does it do?—

It is located within your "enteric nervous system," also known as the "second brain."

Based on its composition, it can significantly influence the following...

→ The parasympathetic/sympathetic nervous system - digest food, absorb and process nutrients (Review week 31)
→ Manage weight and metabolism
→ Your mood, behavior, cognitive performance, stress, and pain tolerance (Review week 31 and 34)
→ Helps your immune system to fight infections and protect against inflammatory disorders, and allergies

—Why is this important?—

Research is recognizing that an imbalance in the microbiome can lead to a host of health problems and inflammatory diseases.

- Inflammatory bowel disease
- Autoimmune disease
- Obesity
- Diabetes
- Heart disease

- Alzheimer's Disease
- Autism Spectrum Disorder
- Anxiety/depression
- Cancer
- and so much more!

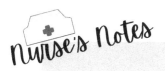

THE GOOD BACTERIA

─So, what do we do?───────────────

Your gut microbiome is shaped by your everyday experiences, and your lifestyle habits can dictate the balance between good and bad bacteria. The goal is to feed the good bacteria to optimize its efficiency, and not let the bad bacteria take over and cause imbalance.

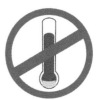

→ **Eat lots of different fruits and vegetables**. The more diverse foods you eat, the more diverse your microbiome is, the healthier you are

→ **Eat lots of whole grains and fiber.** Review week 11 and 15.

→ **Breastfeed for at least 6 months**. Breastfeeding your newborn can establish a healthy microbiome, and is associated with lower rates of allergies, obesity and other health conditions.

───────Top foods with probiotics────────

Yogurt: One of the top sources of probiotics. However, not all yogurt is made equal. Tips:

- Look for yogurt made with active or live cultures

- Low to no sugar added is best, then topped with fresh fruit or honey for added sweetness

- No added sugar plain yogurt is a great substitute for sour cream!

Raw sauerkraut: Not just for your hot dogs. Try it in your burgers or as a side dish to roasted chicken (or another meat dish)!

Kimchi is also a great side to add to your favorite dishes

Sip on **miso soup** as an appetizer

Drink **kefir or kombucha** daily

WEEK 23 CHALLENGE

☆ Update your most common meal list to include your new recent food choices (from week 10)

☆ Discard or hide all junk food in the house

☆ Review M&M Moment

There is a past version of you that is *so proud* of how far you've come!

☆ _____

☆ _____

☆ _____

Sunday

Sleep ☺ 😐 😴

Move your body

Breakfast:

Monday

Sleep ☺ 😐 😴

Move your body

Breakfast:

Tuesday

Sleep ☺ 😐 😴

Move your body

Breakfast:

Wednesday

Sleep 🙂 😐 😴   Breakfast:

Move your body

Thursday

Sleep 🙂 😐 😴   Breakfast:

Move your body

Friday

Sleep 🙂 😐 😴   Breakfast:

Move your body

Saturday

Sleep 🙂 😐 😴   Breakfast:

Move your body

Something I handled well...

FAMILY MEAL PLAN

Breakfast (*On the go!)

_____
_____
_____
_____
_____
_____
_____
_____
_____
_____

Favorite must-have fast food

_____
_____
_____
_____

Designated times fast food is OK!

_____
_____
_____

Lunch/Dinner

_____
_____
_____
_____
_____
_____
_____
_____
_____
_____
_____

Snacks

_____
_____
_____
_____
_____
_____
_____

M&M MOMENT

Challenge: *Discard or hide all junk food in the house*

Out of sight, out of mind. This week, discard or hide all junk food in the house! Your family will be less likely to eat junk food if it is not easily available. If you are the one who purchases and prepares meals, then you are in charge of what you and your family eat. **I empower you** to take this opportunity to cleanse your home of junk food and start fresh. Surround yourself with nutritious foods, and your children will know what's "normal" for your family. From now on, purchase only foods that align with your values for investing in your future health.

Avoid Procrastination

Why do we procrastinate? Simply speaking, making important lifestyle improvements is HARD and the process is stressful. Parenting is already hard enough, and society has given us so many options to make meals "easy, yet junky." But...

There's never going to be a right time, the time is NOW.

Don't compare yourself to anyone, not even your own family who is on the same journey as you! YOU and your body can work WITH time to give you the best long healthy life you deserve. "Healthy" looks different for everyone. Define what works for your family.

The reality is, people nowadays are living longer lives due to medical advancements, but we are spending that latter part of our life going to appointments, taking medications, and prolonging the aging process. It's never too late to reverse or significantly decrease that risk! Remember, being in pursuit of health is now your hobby. Make those significant lifestyle changes, slow the aging process, teach your children the same so you all can FEEL GREAT!

Don't procrastinate. Set your intentions on completing this week's challenges, and conquer them like the mom and pop BOSSES you are!

STRIVE FOR

progress

NOT

perfection

———

PHASE TWO

PUT IT INTO PRACTICE

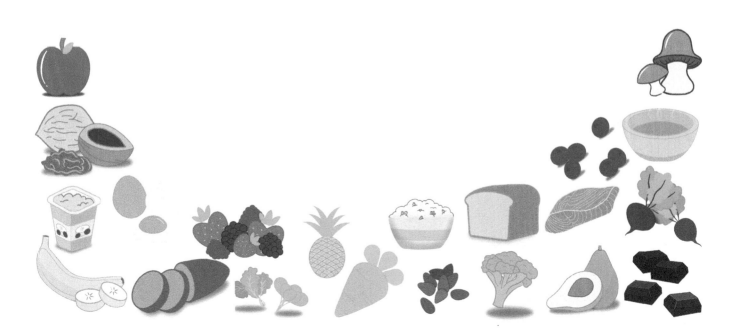

☆ Plan your meals at least 24 hours in advanced to avoid "surprise" stress meals

☐ ☐ ☐ ☐ ☐ ☐ ☐

☆ Review nurse's notes

Eat to
fuel your body,
not feed your
emotions

THIS WEEK'S TOP THREE

☆ _____

☆ _____

☆ _____

Sunday

Sleep ☺ 😐 😴

Move your body

Monday

Sleep ☺ 😐 😴

Move your body

Tuesday

Sleep ☺ 😐 😴

Move your body

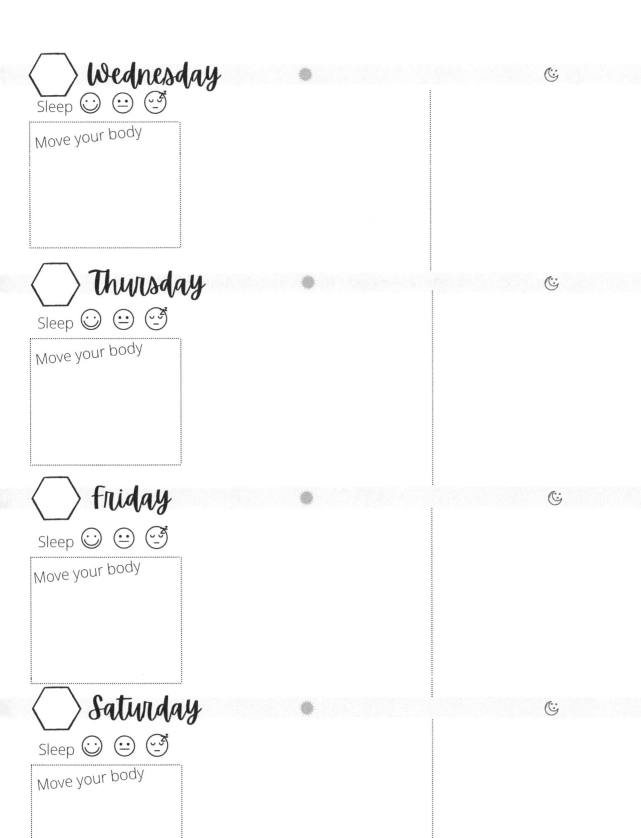

Wednesday

Sleep 🙂 😐 😴

Move your body

Thursday

Sleep 🙂 😐 😴

Move your body

Friday

Sleep 🙂 😐 😴

Move your body

Saturday

Sleep 🙂 😐 😴

Move your body

A person I appreciated...

M&M MOMENT

Challenge: *Plan all your meals at least 24 hours in advanced to avoid "surprise" stress meals*

You've been doing a wonderful job planning your breakfasts this whole time! Now, step it up, and try planning a whole day's worth of food at least the night before, or if you prefer, plan a whole week in advance. You hopefully have a rough idea of what your week would look like. Use your updated meal plan list from week 23 for reference. Plan your daily **breakfast, snack, lunch, snack, dinner**. Even if you don't end up eating ALL the snacks, it's good to have it as an option, so you don't resort to junk food. Also, learn to love leftovers! They are lifesavers :)

── Things to consider ──

☐ Which day or what time each night you will write out your meal plan?

☐ Which day will you purchase groceries?

☐ Which day(s) this week do we need a quick breakfast to go?

☐ Which day(s) do you have time to prepare breakfast in the morning? Which day(s) can the kids help?

☐ Which day(s) or what time will you prepare your lunches for school/work?

☐ Which day(s) will you have time to prepare dinner? Which day(s) can the kids help?

☐ Which day(s) will require a quick dinner (due to picking up kids late from after-school activities, potentially working overtime)?

☐ Is there a special occasion this week? (birthday, big test on Friday, project completed at work, or simply - it's our weekly popcorn, ice cream, and movie night)

*Make copies of the weekly meal plan and post it on the fridge so everyone knows what foods are available!

Weekly Meal Plan

SUNDAY

B:

L:

D:

S:

S:

☐ Water
☐☐ 2 servings fruit
☐☐☐ 3 servings veggies
☐☐☐ Balanced carb
and protiein each meal

MONDAY

B:

L:

D:

S:

S:

☐ Water
☐☐ 2 servings fruit
☐☐☐ 3 servings veggies
☐☐☐ Balanced carb
and protein each meal

TUESDAY

B:

L:

D:

S:

S:

☐ Water
☐☐ 2 servings fruit
☐☐☐ 3 servings veggies
☐☐☐ Balanced carb
and protein each meal

WEDNESDAY

B:

L:

D:

S:

S:

☐ Water
☐☐ 2 servings fruit
☐☐☐ 3 servings veggies
☐☐☐ Balanced carb
and protein each meal

THURSDAY

B:

L:

D:

S:

S:

☐ Water
☐☐ 2 servings fruit
☐☐☐ 3 servings veggies
☐☐☐ Balanced carb
and protein each meal

FRIDAY

B:

L:

D:

S:

S:

☐ Water
☐☐ 2 servings fruit
☐☐☐ 3 servings veggies
☐☐☐ Balanced carb
and protein each meal

SATURDAY

B:

L:

D:

S:

S:

☐ Water
☐☐ 2 servings fruit
☐☐☐ 3 servings veggies
☐☐☐ Balanced carb
and protein each meal

GROCERY LIST

☆ Continue to practice planning your meals at least 24 hours in advanced

☐ ☐ ☐ ☐ ☐ ☐ ☐

☆ Review M&M Moments

JUNK FOOD YOU CRAVED FOR AN HOUR, OR THE BODY AND HEALTH YOU CRAVED FOR A LIFETIME?

THIS WEEK'S TOP THREE

☆ _____

☆ _____

☆ _____

Sunday

Sleep 🙂 😐 😴

Move your body

Monday

Sleep 🙂 😐 😴

Move your body

Tuesday

Sleep 🙂 😐 😴

Move your body

Wednesday

Sleep 🙂 😐 😴

Move your body

Thursday

Sleep 🙂 😐 😴

Move your body

Friday

Sleep 🙂 😐 😴

Move your body

Saturday

Sleep 🙂 😐 😴

Move your body

I am proud of myself for...

M&M MOMENT

80/20 rule

There have been SO many new rules and guidelines introduced these last several months, it's easy to get overwhelmed! But remember, **perfection is the enemy of progress.** These rules and guidelines are #goals to keep in mind, but always allow yourself some flexibility. The word "diet" makes us feel deprived, which risks putting you on a slippery slope to splurging and overeating. The 80/20 rule is a great idea to start with and eventually work towards a 90/10 rule. This means 80% of the time, you eat whole, mostly unprocessed, nutritious foods, and 20% of the time can be whatever you want as long as it was planned for. Nothing is off-limits. It helps you to maintain a balanced mindset about eating, removing emotional attachments, such as guilt and stress to food. Instead of thinking about what you can't eat (restrictive mindset), practice moderation so you can fit in all the good foods you learned about (abundance mindset).

3 meals (breakfast, lunch, dinner) x 7 days = 21 meals
20% = 4 meals

If seeing a number makes you anxious, remember you still have control and you define what "occasional" foods mean to your family! The priority is always to do better than yesterday.

Mental note: It's important to not label your meals as "rewards" or "punishments." Food is meant to nourish your body AND be pleasurable. So enjoy your 20% "cheat meals," because it is a part of your diet, embrace it!

 Which foods make the 20% cut? When do you plan to enjoy these foods?

_____   _____

_____   _____

_____   _____

Managing decision fatigue

With all the micro-decisions you make every day, food seems to be an easy one to cheat yourself out of. This is a huge BARRIER. Some excuses that come up...

- ✗ I'm not in the mood for this food today
- ✗ I don't want leftovers
- ✗ I don't have the energy to prepare this meal
- ✗ I have lots of energy today, I want to cook something fabulous!
- ✗ I'm bored of this, I want to try something new

So, what do you do?

- ✓ Give yourself GRACE. Don't apologize for how you feel and instead explore those feelings
- ✓ Remember what you eat and drink is simply created to provide nutrients and energy for your body to function, not just for pleasure
- ✓ Don't think too hard! You don't have to come up with brand new meals every time, experiment "healthifying" your family's favorite meals
- ✓ If all fails, plan for your favorite fast food meal!

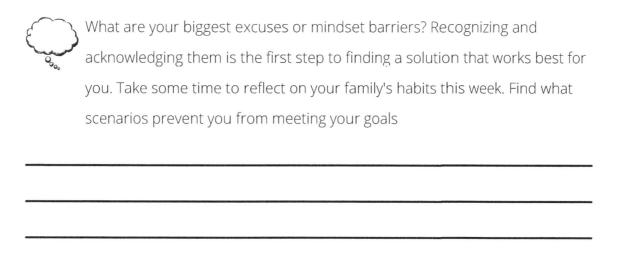 What are your biggest excuses or mindset barriers? Recognizing and acknowledging them is the first step to finding a solution that works best for you. Take some time to reflect on your family's habits this week. Find what scenarios prevent you from meeting your goals

_____

_____

_____

_____

_____

☆ Send a message to someone each day to express your gratitude.

☐ ☐ ☐ ☐ ☐ ☐ ☐

☆ Pick a challenge from previous weeks. Finding a healthier alternative or adding a serving of nutrients?

NOTE TO SELF: WHEN I EAT LIKE CRAP, I FEEL LIKE CRAP

THIS WEEK'S TOP THREE

☆ _____

☆ _____

☆ _____

Sunday

Sleep ☺ 😐 😴

Move your body

Monday

Sleep ☺ 😐 😴

Move your body

Tuesday

Sleep ☺ 😐 😴

Move your body

Wednesday

Sleep 🙂 😐 😴

Move your body

Thursday

Sleep 🙂 😐 😴

Move your body

Friday

Sleep 🙂 😐 😴

Move your body

Saturday

Sleep 🙂 😐 😴

Move your body

Something that brought me joy...

6 MONTH REFLECTION

☆ What were your family's biggest accomplishments?

☆ What were your biggest fears/stressors?

☆ How did you or do you plan on overcoming those fears/stressors?

☆ Have you noticed any changes in your family, such as behavior, symptoms or etc.?

☆ The funniest thing that happened was...

☆ We're one step closer to our goals because...

KID'S TIME TO SHINE

Space for your kids to write or draw what they enjoyed the most this last month

MONTHLY HABIT TRACKER

Print one out for each family member & post it on your family board! Track the habits you are concentrating on. Color it in after completing it and celebrate every day's win! 1 symbol = 1 day.

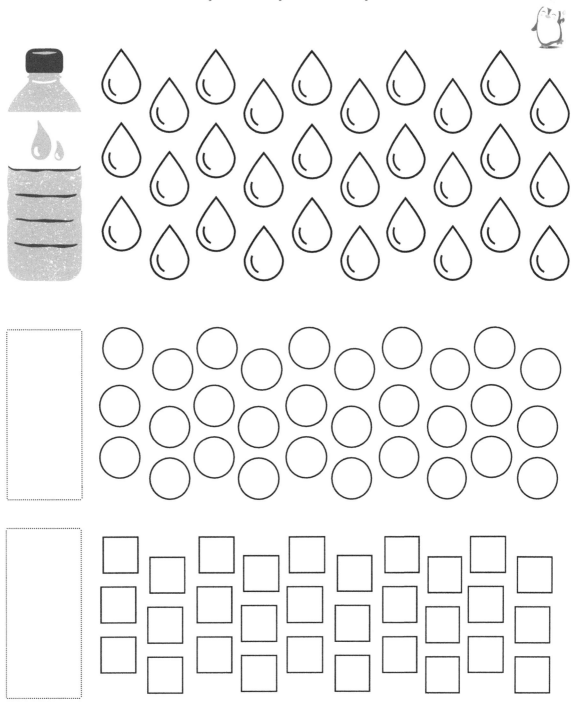

WEEK 27 CHALLENGE

☆ Congratulations on surviving 6 months - you're half way there!

☆ Plan one day this week to DRESS UP and treat your family to something special

☆ Complete 6 month reflection & vision board

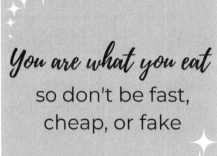

You are what you eat so don't be fast, cheap, or fake

THIS WEEK'S TOP THREE

☆ _____

☆ _____

☆ _____

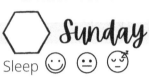 **Sunday**

Sleep 🙂 😐 😴

Move your body

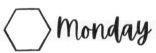 **Monday**

Sleep 🙂 😐 😴

Move your body

Tuesday

Sleep 🙂 😐 😴

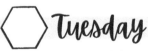

Move your body

Wednesday

Sleep 🙂 😐 😴

Move your body

Thursday

Sleep 🙂 😐 😴

Move your body

Friday

Sleep 🙂 😐 😴

Move your body

Saturday

Sleep 🙂 😐 😴

Move your body

Something that brought me joy...

VISION BOARD

6 MONTH CHALLENGE: UPDATE YOUR VISION BOARD. Draw, print, or use pictures from a magazine. Fill this page with your family's favorite things that make you happy and stay motivated. Ex. pictures of loved ones, pets, dream vacation, hobbies, favorite things, etc.

CREATIVE SPACE

You will have "off days." Look back on these pages to remind you why you started this journey!

VISION BOARD

Reaching the "ultimate goal" is not a final destination, it is something that you make the conscious decision to achieve every day in your life. You'll look back years from now and realize how far you have come!

Use this space to define what makes YOU and your family feel healthy and accomplished. What are your family's unique needs? Consider: your family's health, your children's school grades, your family's behavior, how you handle stressors - the big and small things, your productivity at home and work, your finances, etc. Clean eating can do wonders on all of this! Dig deep and DREAM BIG.

WEEK 28 CHALLENGE

☆ Welcome to your 21-day clean eating challenge!

☆ Recognize patterns in your family's behaviors and physical symptoms related to food

☆ Find your favorite influence on YouTube/IG/FB and learn new recipes!

The distance between your dreams and reality is called *Action*

THIS WEEK'S TOP THREE

☆ _____

☆ _____

☆ _____

Sunday

Sleep 🙂 😐 😴

Move your body

Monday

Sleep 🙂 😐 😴

Move your body

Tuesday

Sleep 🙂 😐 😴

Move your body

Wednesday

Sleep 🙂 😐 😣

Move your body

Thursday

Sleep 🙂 😐 😣

Move your body

Friday

Sleep 🙂 😐 😣

Move your body

Saturday

Sleep 🙂 😐 😣

Move your body

A favorite memory that always make me smile...

21 DAY CLEAN EATING CHALLENGE

You have been challenged to add more foods to your diet and swap out foods that included the "forbidden four" for cleaner versions. This helps switch you from a restrictive mindset to food abundance. You have also been practicing your meal planning. You are doing an amazing job!! So let's step it up and put it all together! The next 21 days will challenge you a little different because we will be emphasizing what NOT to eat, but hoping you don't lose sight of all the new foods you learned you CAN eat! I know we just learned about the 80/20 rule, but even this rule is voided for 21 days. What's the goal? ***To cleanse your body from added sugars and processed chemicals.***

Benefits

⭐ You will FEEL GREAT!! It's always hard at first, but you won't regret it!

⭐ You will have more energy

⭐ You will have less brain fog and more focus

⭐ You will be less irritable

⭐ You will learn what your mind and body are capable of

⭐ This is your chance to see firsthand how your body reacts to food

Reminders

✓ Plan your meals at least 24 hours in advance - breakfast, lunch, dinner, and 2 snacks available

✓ Do not skip your meals! Try to eat every 3-4 hours to keep your blood sugar stable and your brain and body fueled

✓ Review weeks 6 and 7 to freshen up on portion control and hunger cues

✓ Don't forget to drink enough water for your body weight DAILY! (Week 4)

✓ Use Master Weekly Plan to post on your fridge or Healthy Habits Board

✓ Make copies of the individual "Food and Habit Tracker" for each family member to measure progress

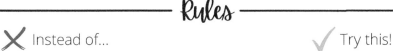

Rules

✗ Instead of...	✓ Try this!
Soda, juices, energy drinks	Water, blended whole fruit juices, smoothies
Coffee or tea with sweeteners	Try it plain! You'll get the full benefits of antioxidants found in coffee and tea without the sweeteners
Fried foods	Baked foods covered with whole wheat panko for added crunch (no added sugar)
Highly processed packaged snacks	Look for snacks with minimal ingredients that do not include the "forbidden four"
White breads, pastas, rice, tortillas	Look for WHOLE grains, brown rice, and nothing with added sugars
Processed meats with added sugars/nitrites	Look for bacon or sausage that are UNCURED, NO nitrites, and NO sugar

Ultimate rule: Cut out all foods with "forbidden four" and "added sugars"

 M&M MOMENT

Challenge: *Recognize patterns in your behavior and physical symptom related to food*

Get to know your body more intimately by tracking your elimination patterns, behavior, and physical symptoms. This empowers you and your family to learn how food impacts your bodies. Some kids can't distinguish between having a stomachache from illness, cramping for bowel movement, or simply being full after eating. Help them learn to describe their feelings so they can communicate their needs better. This Food and Symptom Tracker includes space to explore and write in these symptoms. Start with a "before" assessment, and complete it at least once a week to discover an overall pattern. There's also space to write notes each day as needed. Make copies of the symptom tracker (found in week 31) for each family member.

Keep in mind that this is to introduce mind-body awareness related to food, not to diagnose any medical conditions. If you find you have concerns or sensitivity to foods, speak with your doctor more about it.

Weekly Food & Habit Tracker

KNOW YOUR BODY

Bowel Movements
   Loose | Soft/Normal | Hard
   Irregular | Regular Pattern
Bloating
   Never | Sometimes | A lot
Cramping or stomachaches
   Never | Sometimes | A lot
Heartburn
   Never | Sometimes | A lot
Headache
   Never | Sometimes | A lot
Itching, rashes, acne
   Never | Sometimes | A lot
Irritable
   Never | Sometimes | A lot
Sluggish
   Never | Sometimes | A lot
Energy Level
   Little | Adequate | Great
Hyperactive
   Never | Sometimes | A lot
Ability to focus
   Hard | OK | Well

SUNDAY
B:
L:
D:
S:
S:

100%!
50%!

Sleep ☺ 😐 😴

MONDAY
B:
L:
D:
S:
S:

100%!
50%!

Sleep ☺ 😐 😴

TUESDAY
B:
L:
D:
S:
S:

100%!
50%!

Sleep ☺ 😐 😴

WEDNESDAY
B:
L:
D:
S:
S:

100%!
50%!

Sleep ☺ 😐 😴

THURSDAY
B:
L:
D:
S:
S:

100%!
50%!

Sleep ☺ 😐 😴

FRIDAY
B:
L:
D:
S:
S:

100%!
50%!

Sleep ☺ 😐 😴

SATURDAY
B:
L:
D:
S:
S:

100%!
50%!

Sleep ☺ 😐 😴

Weekly Food & Habit Tracker

KNOW YOUR BODY

Bowel Movements
   Loose | Soft/Normal | Hard
   Irregular | Regular Pattern
Bloating
   Never | Sometimes | A lot
Cramping or stomachaches
   Never | Sometimes | A lot
Heartburn
   Never | Sometimes | A lot
Headache
   Never | Sometimes | A lot
Itching, rashes, acne
   Never | Sometimes | A lot
Irritable
   Never | Sometimes | A lot
Sluggish
   Never | Sometimes | A lot
Energy Level
   Little | Adequate | Great
Hyperactive
   Never | Sometimes | A lot
Ability to focus
   Hard | OK | Well

SUNDAY
B:
100%!
L:
D: 50%!
S:
S:

Sleep 😊 😐 😴

MONDAY
B:
100%!
L:
D: 50%!
S:
S:

Sleep 😊 😐 😴

TUESDAY
B:
100%!
L:
D: 50%!
S:
S:

Sleep 😊 😐 😴

WEDNESDAY
B:
100%!
L:
D: 50%!
S:
S:

Sleep 😊 😐 😴

THURSDAY
B:
100%!
L:
D: 50%!
S:
S:

Sleep 😊 😐 😴

FRIDAY
B:
100%!
L:
D: 50%!
S:
S:

Sleep 😊 😐 😴

SATURDAY
B:
100%!
L:
D: 50%!
S:
S:

Sleep 😊 😐 😴

MONTHLY REFLECTION

Use this time to review your vision board and update as needed!

☆ A moment I can't forget...

☆ The hardest thing about this past month was...

☆ We got through the hardest times together by...

☆ I am so proud of...

☆ Best meal I thouroughly enjoyed:

☆ The funniest thing that happened was...

KID'S TIME TO SHINE

Space for your kids to write or draw what they enjoyed the most this last month

MONTHLY HABIT TRACKER

Print one out for each family member & post it on your family board! Track the habits you are concentrating on. Color it in after completing it and celebrate every day's win! 1 symbol = 1 day.

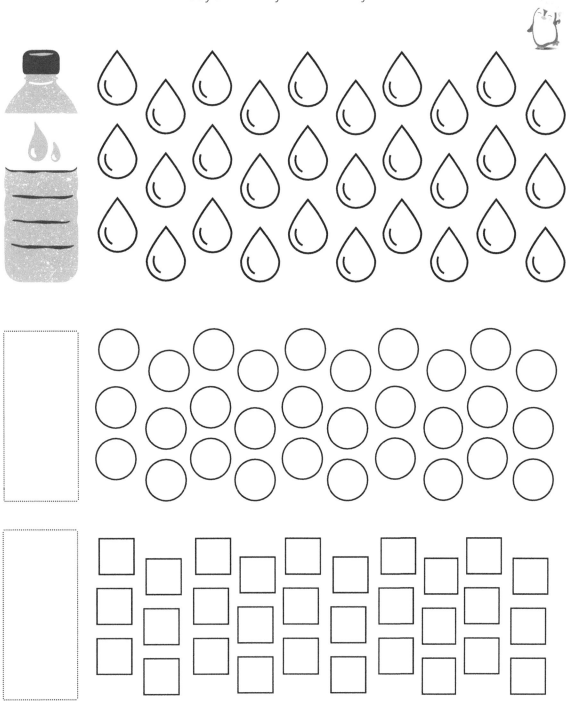

☆ Continue 21 Day Challenge!

☐ ☐ ☐ ☐ ☐ ☐ ☐

☆ Drink a smoothie or blended juice for at least 5 days this week!

☐ ☐ ☐ ☐ ☐ ☐ ☐

☆ Review M&M Moment

Nothing looks as good as *healthy feels!*

THIS WEEK'S TOP THREE

☆ _____

☆ _____

☆ _____

⬡ **Sunday**

Sleep 🙂 😐 😫

Move your body

⬡ **Monday**

Sleep 🙂 😐 😫

Move your body

⬡ **Tuesday**

Sleep 🙂 😐 😫

Move your body

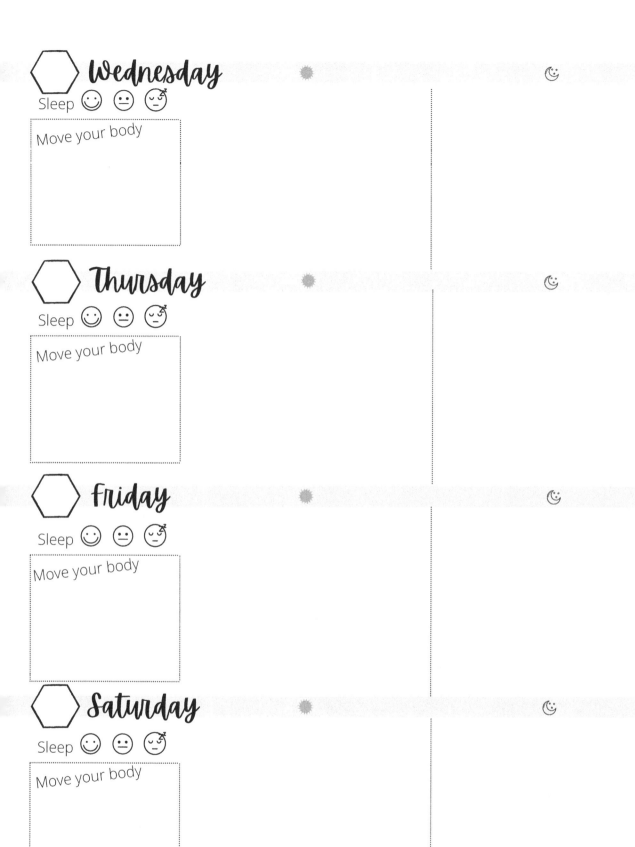

Wednesday

Sleep 🙂 😐 😴

Move your body

Thursday

Sleep 🙂 😐 😴

Move your body

Friday

Sleep 🙂 😐 😴

Move your body

Saturday

Sleep 🙂 😐 😴

Move your body

I am thankful for...

Remember - health and wellness is a journey, not a destination

When you consciously make the decision to begin your journey to health and wellness, you are making a long-term promise to yourself. You are in pursuit of health, making the best decisions you can each day to invest in a healthier tomorrow. But you are human. And during this journey, you will make mistakes, you will have cravings, and you will have off days. That is OK. It's unrealistic to expect yourself to be consistent every moment, every day, forever, from now on. But do not throw all your hard work and healthy habits out the window because of ANYTHING. Life will happen. Significant life events will happen. These are out of your control. What is ALWAYS in your control, is the decision you make to nourish your body for health.

Cravings

With that being said, let's talk about CRAVINGS.

Up until now, you have been living in a state of abundance. Now you are taking a step into completely eliminating sugar on top of the "forbidden four" for these 21 days. Cravings and temptations may sneak up on you. _Just for these 21 days, DON'T DO IT!_

- Food cravings happen, you can't control your mind or emotions from wanting something, but you CAN control your reaction to it
- By refusing to give in to your cravings, you are taking power from it and taking control of your meals
- YOU say when you will have a piece of that cake. Don't let your emotions or situation dictate what you eat

After these 21 days, that's another story. PLAN FOR IT. If ice cream is your favorite treat, plan to have ice cream after a long day of work on Fridays after lunch. Do it unapologetically and enjoy it wholeheartedly because you know you were in control and you deserve it!

Weekly Food & Habit Tracker

KNOW YOUR BODY

Bowel Movements
    Loose | Soft/Normal | Hard
    Irregular | Regular Pattern
Bloating
    Never | Sometimes | A lot
Cramping or stomachaches
    Never | Sometimes | A lot
Heartburn
    Never | Sometimes | A lot
Headache
    Never | Sometimes | A lot
Itching, rashes, acne
    Never | Sometimes | A lot
Irritable
    Never | Sometimes | A lot
Sluggish
    Never | Sometimes | A lot
Energy Level
    Little | Adequate | Great
Hyperactive
    Never | Sometimes | A lot
Ability to focus
    Hard | OK | Well

SUNDAY

B: 100%!

L:

D: 50%!

S:

S:

Sleep 😊 😐 😴

MONDAY

B: 100%!

L:

D: 50%!

S:

S:

Sleep 😊 😐 😴

TUESDAY

B: 100%!

L:

D: 50%!

S:

S:

Sleep 😊 😐 😴

WEDNESDAY

B: 100%!

L:

D: 50%!

S:

S:

Sleep 😊 😐 😴

THURSDAY

B: 100%!

L:

D: 50%!

S:

S:

Sleep 😊 😐 😴

FRIDAY

B: 100%!

L:

D: 50%!

S:

S:

Sleep 😊 😐 😴

SATURDAY

B: 100%!

L:

D: 50%!

S:

S:

Sleep 😊 😐 😴

☆ Continue 21 day food
   challenge!

☐ ☐ ☐ ☐ ☐ ☐ ☐

☆ Herbal teas have many health
   benefits! Find a tea you all can
   enjoy every day. Our favorite
   is Red Rooibos. It's caffeine-
   free and high in antioxidants!

Be stronger
than your excuses

THIS WEEK'S TOP THREE

☆ _____

☆ _____

_____

☆ _____

_____

⬡ **Sunday**

Sleep 😊 😐 😴

Move your body

⬡ **Monday**

Sleep 😊 😐 😴

Move your body

⬡ **Tuesday**

Sleep 😊 😐 😴

Move your body

Wednesday

Sleep 🙂 😐 😴

Move your body

Thursday

Sleep 🙂 😐 😴

Move your body

Friday

Sleep 🙂 😐 😴

Move your body

Saturday

Sleep 🙂 😐 😴

Move your body

Something I handled well...

Weekly Food & Habit Tracker

KNOW YOUR BODY

Bowel Movements
   Loose | Soft/Normal | Hard
   Irregular | Regular Pattern
Bloating
   Never | Sometimes | A lot
Cramping or stomachaches
   Never | Sometimes | A lot
Heartburn
   Never | Sometimes | A lot
Headache
   Never | Sometimes | A lot
Itching, rashes, acne
   Never | Sometimes | A lot
Irritable
   Never | Sometimes | A lot
Sluggish
   Never | Sometimes | A lot
Energy Level
   Little | Adequate | Great
Hyperactive
   Never | Sometimes | A lot
Ability to focus
   Hard | OK | Well

SUNDAY
B:
L:
D:
S:
S:
100%!
50%!
Sleep ☺ 😐 😴

MONDAY
B:
L:
D:
S:
S:
100%!
50%!
Sleep ☺ 😐 😴

TUESDAY
B:
L:
D:
S:
S:
100%!
50%!
Sleep ☺ 😐 😴

WEDNESDAY
B:
L:
D:
S:
S:
100%!
50%!
Sleep ☺ 😐 😴

THURSDAY
B:
L:
D:
S:
S:
100%!
50%!
Sleep ☺ 😐 😴

FRIDAY
B:
L:
D:
S:
S:
100%!
50%!
Sleep ☺ 😐 😴

SATURDAY
B:
L:
D:
S:
S:
100%!
50%!
Sleep ☺ 😐 😴

Weekly Food & Habit Tracker

KNOW YOUR BODY

Bowel Movements
   Loose | Soft/Normal | Hard
   Irregular | Regular Pattern
Bloating
   Never | Sometimes | A lot
Cramping or stomachaches
   Never | Sometimes | A lot
Heartburn
   Never | Sometimes | A lot
Headache
   Never | Sometimes | A lot
Itching, rashes, acne
   Never | Sometimes | A lot
Irritable
   Never | Sometimes | A lot
Sluggish
   Never | Sometimes | A lot
Energy Level
   Little | Adequate | Great
Hyperactive
   Never | Sometimes | A lot
Ability to focus
   Hard | OK | Well

SUNDAY
B:
L:
D:
S:
S:
100%!
50%!

Sleep 😊 😐 😴

MONDAY
B:
L:
D:
S:
S:
100%!
50%!

Sleep 😊 😐 😴

TUESDAY
B:
L:
D:
S:
S:
100%!
50%!

Sleep 😊 😐 😴

WEDNESDAY
B:
L:
D:
S:
S:
100%!
50%!

Sleep 😊 😐 😴

THURSDAY
B:
L:
D:
S:
S:
100%!
50%!

Sleep 😊 😐 😴

FRIDAY
B:
L:
D:
S:
S:
100%!
50%!

Sleep 😊 😐 😴

SATURDAY
B:
L:
D:
S:
S:
100%!
50%!

Sleep 😊 😐 😴

WEEK 31 CHALLENGE

☆ Congratulations on completing your 21 day clean eating challenge! Plan a date to treat your family something special

☆ Complete another "Know Your Body" Assessment and reflection

Create
Healthy habits,
not restrictions

THIS WEEK'S TOP THREE

☆ _____

☆ _____

☆ _____

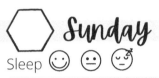 **Sunday**

Sleep 🙂 😐 😴

Move your body

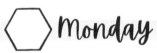 **Monday**

Sleep 🙂 😐 😴

Move your body

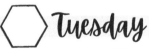 **Tuesday**

Sleep 🙂 😐 😴

Move your body

Wednesday

Sleep 😊 😐 😴

Move your body

Thursday

Sleep 😊 😐 😴

Move your body

Friday

Sleep 😊 😐 😴

Move your body

Saturday

Sleep 😊 😐 😴

Move your body

A person I appreciated...

21 DAY CHALLENGE REFLECTION

☆ What did you notice about your elimination patterns and physical symptoms? Worsened, improved, stayed the same?

☆ Which of your favorite foods and/or ingredient were the hardest to eliminate or which rule was the hardest to follow?

☆ How did you or do you plan on overcoming those fears/stressors?

☆ Which food did you miss & plan on adding it to your OK list in 80/20 rule?

☆ Which foods did you realize you can live without?

☆ I am so proud of...

21 DAY CHALLENGE REFLECTION

KNOW YOUR BODY

Bowel Movements
  Loose | Soft/Normal | Hard
  Irregular | Regular Pattern
Bloating
  Never | Sometimes | A lot
Cramping or stomachaches
  Never | Sometimes | A lot
Heartburn
  Never | Sometimes | A lot
Headache
  Never | Sometimes | A lot
Itching, rashes, acne
  Never | Sometimes | A lot
Irritable
  Never | Sometimes | A lot
Sluggish
  Never | Sometimes | A lot
Energy Level
  Little | Adequate | Great
Hyperactive
  Never | Sometimes | A lot
Ability to focus
  Hard | OK | Well

KNOW YOUR BODY

Bowel Movements
  Loose | Soft/Normal | Hard
  Irregular | Regular Pattern
Bloating
  Never | Sometimes | A lot
Cramping or stomachaches
  Never | Sometimes | A lot
Heartburn
  Never | Sometimes | A lot
Headache
  Never | Sometimes | A lot
Itching, rashes, acne
  Never | Sometimes | A lot
Irritable
  Never | Sometimes | A lot
Sluggish
  Never | Sometimes | A lot
Energy Level
  Little | Adequate | Great
Hyperactive
  Never | Sometimes | A lot
Ability to focus
  Hard | OK | Well

- Make copies of this for each family member
- Complete one before the 21-day challenge, at least once a week, and at the end of the 21 days.
- Complete again as needed after reintroducing foods that you have previously eliminated

*Reintroducing foods after not eating it for 3 weeks may cause behavior or physical symptoms. Pay attention to it! This may mean you are sensitive to the food. Consider cutting down or eliminating based on level of discomfort. Questions? Ask your doctor. Otherwise, enjoy!

THE
Happiness
OF YOUR LIFE
DEPENDS ON THE
Quality
OF YOUR
THOUGHTS

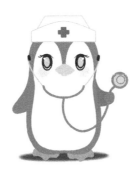

PHASE THREE

STRESS

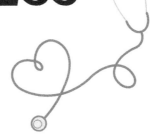

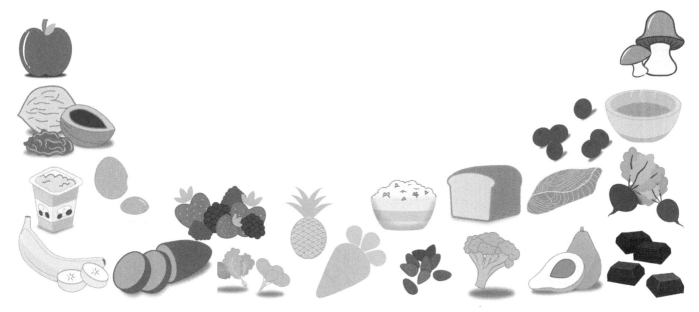

☆ Review nurse's notes

☆ Drink your water daily!

☐ ☐ ☐ ☐ ☐ ☐ ☐

☆ Update meal list as needed

Never lose hope in the body's ability to *Heal itself*

☆ _____

☆ _____

☆ _____

Sunday

Sleep 😊 😐 😣

Move your body

Monday

Sleep 😊 😐 😣

Move your body

Tuesday

Sleep 😊 😐 😣

Move your body

Wednesday

Sleep 🙂 😐 😴

Move your body

Thursday

Sleep 🙂 😐 😴

Move your body

Friday

Sleep 🙂 😐 😴

Move your body

Saturday

Sleep 🙂 😐 😴

Move your body

Something new I learned this week...

INVEST IN YOUR HEALTH - REMINDERS

☐ Does your family constantly get sick with colds or the flu?

☐ Are you battling fatigue, headaches, anxiety, depression, or trouble sleeping?

☐ Do you have digestive problems such as stomachaches, acid reflux, constipation?

These are just a few symptoms that come from poor daily habits causing an imbalance in your hormones and metabolism. As you age, your body undergoes the natural wear and tear of everyday life, but your ability to regenerate itself decreases.

#1 Food is one of the most important ingredients you need for good health. That is why learning about food makes up the bulk of this planner. The primary goal is to provide resources to help you make educated decisions daily that will decrease risks of the above symptoms, prevent disease, delay the aging process, and make a positive impact on your health long-term. This can be done by eating the right foods. Feeding your body with the right nutrients will help heal, repair, and rebuild itself. Don't lose sight of everything you have learned! Review the weekly challenges often for reminders.

The next lifestyle challenge that's worth tackling is your reactions to stress. Stress has become an inevitable part of a busy life. Stress is difficult to eliminate, but there are ways to help bring your body back to a state of calm in the midst of stress. This state of calm gives it time to replenish your body's resources to make decisions without fatigue or brain fog and tackle life's challenges.

Whole Health

PHYSICAL, EMOTIONAL, NUTRITIONAL, ENVIRONMENTAL, AND SPIRITUAL

You will realize that everything is connected to everything. If one part of your foundation is unstable, it causes instability in the other pillars. Taking care of all these aspects in your life is the epitome of self-care. Give yourself and your family the gift of health and keep it going. If you have made it this far, you're doing amazing!

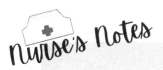

STRESS

Stress is an inevitable part of life. But did you know that constant stress can be detrimental to your health? Stress comes in many shapes and forms. Some examples include...

- Nutritional stress: alcohol, **sugar, inflammatory foods, skipping meals, low-calorie diets, insufficient nutrients**

- Physical stress: **lack of uninterrupted sleep**, overexercising, smoking

- Emotional stress: anxiety, family, trauma, work, financial, family, school

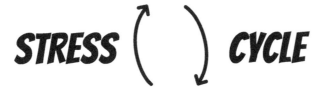

STRESS ( ) **CYCLE**

✗ Causes imbalance of hormones, which leads to **difficulty sleeping**, fatigue, and anxiety
✗ **Decrease absorption of nutrients, malnourished,** indigestion
✗ Increase fat storage ~> gain weight and increase risk of diabetes or obesity
✗ Muscle tension that can lead to headaches and generalized aches and pains
✗ Risk of high blood pressure, **inflammation**, and other chronic diseases

Notice HOW AND WHAT WE EAT and HOW MUCH WE SLEEP causes more nutritional and sleep problems in our body? When you're stressed, your body is not releasing the right hormones to digest your food efficiently which can lead to the inability to absorb the nutrition from all the healthy foods you've been eating. The lack of nutrients is stressful to your body, causing the cycle to repeat. It's this constant cycle that needs to be broken.

───────────── *Stress-busting foods* ─────────────

Superfood highlight: Blueberries and dark chocolate are high in antioxidants that are perfect foods for the brain. Also, review Omega 3's in week 19 and Balanced Breakfast in week 11 for more about brain foods

MONTHLY REFLECTION

Use this time to review your vision board and update as needed!

☆ What were your family's biggest accomplishments?

☆ What were your biggest fears/stressors?

☆ How did you or do you plan on overcoming those fears/stressors?

☆ Have you noticed any changes in your family, such as behavior, symptoms or etc.?

☆ Best meal I thouroughly enjoyed:

☆ The funniest thing that happened was...

KID'S TIME TO SHINE

Space for your kids to write or draw what they enjoyed the most this last month

MONTHLY HABIT TRACKER

Print one out for each family member & post it on your family board! Track the habits you are concentrating on. Color it in after completing it and celebrate every day's win! 1 symbol = 1 day.

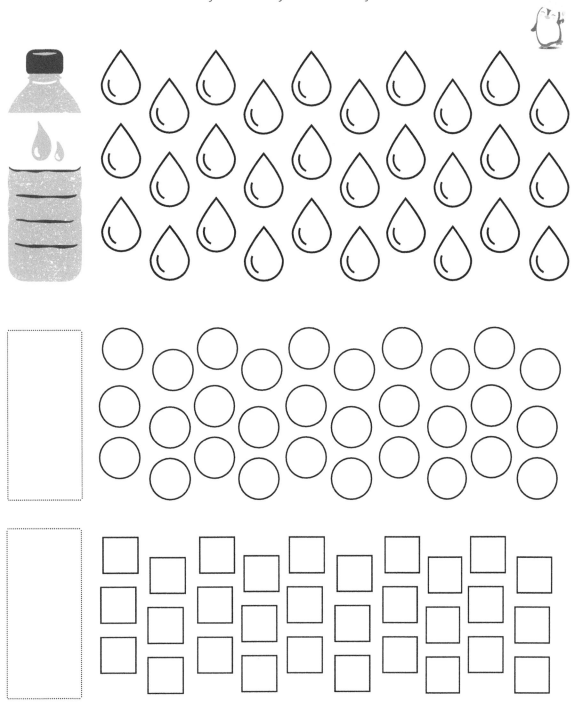

WEEK 33 CHALLENGE

☆ Discover your stressors

☆ Are you still eating 2 servings
   of fruit daily?
   ☐ ☐ ☐ ☐ ☐ ☐ ☐

> ONCE YOU REPLACE
> NEGATIVE THOUGHTS
> WITH POSITIVE ONES,
> YOU'LL START HAVING
> POSITIVE RESULTS
>
> – WILLIE NELSON

THIS WEEK'S TOP THREE

☆ _____

☆ _____

☆ _____

⬡ Sunday

Sleep 🙂 😐 😫

Move your body

⬡ Monday

Sleep 🙂 😐 😫

Move your body

⬡ Tuesday

Sleep 🙂 😐 😫

Move your body

Wednesday

Sleep 🙂 😐 😫

Move your body

Thursday

Sleep 🙂 😐 😫

Move your body

Friday

Sleep 🙂 😐 😫

Move your body

Saturday

Sleep 🙂 😐 😫

Move your body

I am proud of myself for...

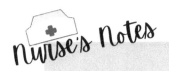

STRESS

Challenge: *Discover your stressors*

What types of unresolved long-term stress do you and your family struggle with? Recognizing and acknowledging it is the first step in finding the right solutions that work best for your family! It's unrealistic to eliminate the stressors, but it is important to give your body time for relaxation to maintain balance, even for a moment. You will learn small simple changes to help manage some of these stressors. **Hint: If you are not sleeping well or eating well, your brain does not have the capacity or balance in hormones to manage stress effectively**

STRESSORS I CAN CONTROL

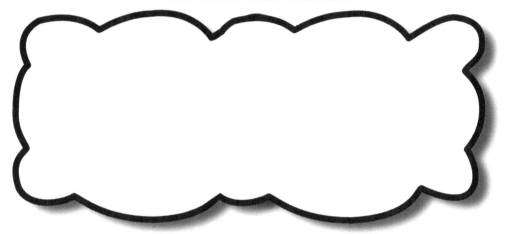

STRESSORS I CANNOT CONTROL

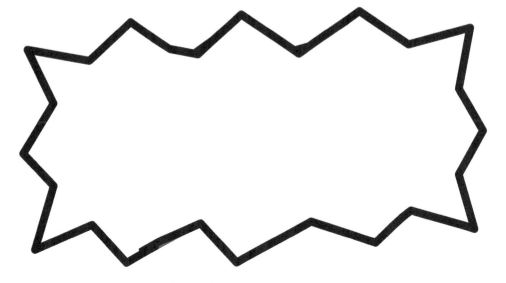

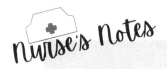

THE PROBLEM WITH STRESS

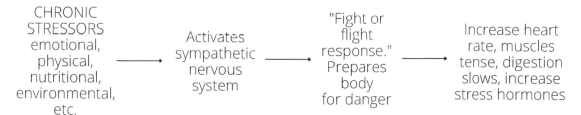

CHRONIC STRESSORS emotional, physical, nutritional, environmental, etc. → Activates sympathetic nervous system → "Fight or flight response." Prepares body for danger → Increase heart rate, muscles tense, digestion slows, increase stress hormones

Chronic stress is similar to a car that's always running without proper maintenance, it will break down faster. Stress puts a toll on your bodies. Harvard shares in an article that "Over time, repeated activation of the stress response takes a toll on the body. Research suggests that chronic stress contributes to **high blood pressure, promotes the formation of artery-clogging deposits, and causes brain changes that may contribute to anxiety, depression, and addiction..** More preliminary research suggests that chronic stress may also contribute to obesity, both through direct mechanisms (causing people to eat more) or indirectly (decreasing sleep and exercise)."

Understanding the stress response. 2020. Harvard Health Publishing. https://www.health.harvard.edu/staying-healthy/understanding-the-stress-response

So, what do we do?

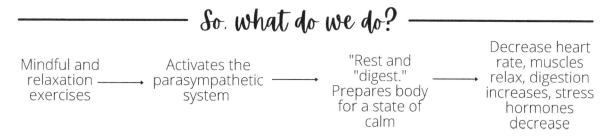

Mindful and relaxation exercises → Activates the parasympathetic system → "Rest and "digest." Prepares body for a state of calm → Decrease heart rate, muscles relax, digestion increases, stress hormones decrease

Strengthen and activate your parasympathetic system

Fresh outdoor air

Deep breathing

Laughter

Stretching

Massage

Meditation

Your favorite hobby

Positive thoughts

Short walk outside

SLEEP

Be mindful about the present

Warm bath

Prayer

Music

Visualization

Slow down - Don't multitask

Yoga, qi gong, tai chi

Journaling

Positive conversation

Decrease caffeine and sugar

WEEK 34 CHALLENGE

☆ Google your favorite mantras and say these OUT LOUD upon waking

☐ ☐ ☐ ☐ ☐ ☐ ☐

☆ Practice Deep Breathing at least twice a day

☐ ☐ ☐ ☐ ☐ ☐ ☐

☆ Kid's time to shine activity

HEALING DOESN'T MEAN THE DAMAGE NEVER EXISTED. IT MEANS THE DAMAGE NO LONGER CONTROLS YOUR LIFE

– AKSHAY DUBBED

THIS WEEK'S TOP THREE

☆ _____

☆ _____

☆ _____

Sunday

Sleep 😊 😐 😴

Move your body

Monday

Sleep 😊 😐 😴

Move your body

Tuesday

Sleep 😊 😐 😴

Move your body

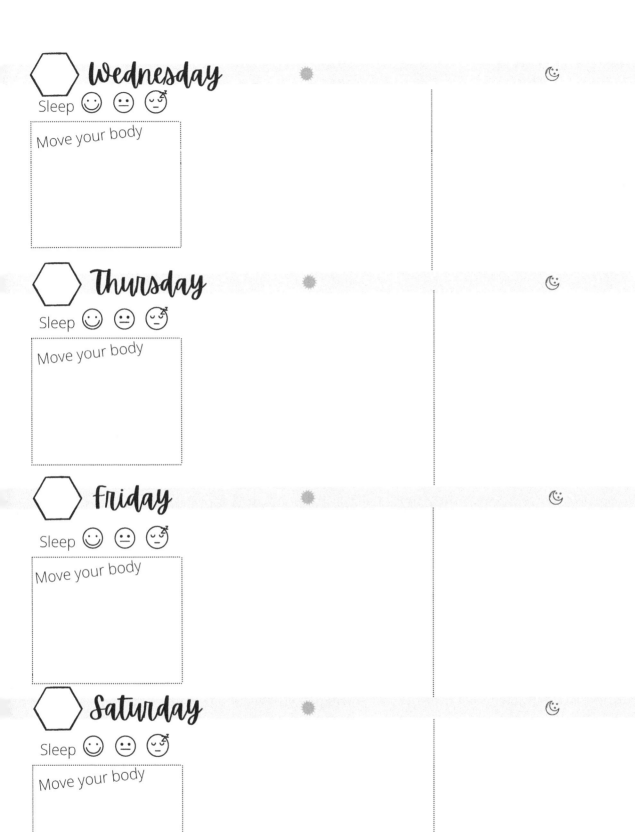

Wednesday

Sleep 🙂 😐 😴

Move your body

Thursday

Sleep 🙂 😐 😴

Move your body

Friday

Sleep 🙂 😐 😴

Move your body

Saturday

Sleep 🙂 😐 😴

Move your body

Something that brough me joy...

STRESS IN CHILDREN

It's important to recognize that stress in children may look different. Sometimes stress can be displayed as emotional or physical problems and can be subtle at first. You know your kids best! If anything seems unusual to you, intervene!

- Upset stomach
- Headaches
- Nightmares
- Trouble sleeping
- Trouble concentrating
- Decreased motivation
- New fears
- Body insecurities

- Changes in eating habits
- Bedwetting
- Doesn't want to participate in activities
- Restlessness
- Regressing towards comforting behaviors from their younger selves - thumbsucking, nail-biting

So, what do you do?

It's also important to recognize that a toddler's tantrum is a form of releasing their stress and "big emotions." They physiologically cannot control it on their own. Teaching toddlers and kids to be resilient and how to manage stress at a young age can benefit them for life, so they will not succumb to such mental or physical problems that we suffer as adults. Here are some basic ideas to get started with...

→ Acknowledge their feelings, listen to them without giving advice or being critical

→ Create a safe, positive environment, give them a sense of control

→ Monitor activities, TV shows, or games, avoid anything controversial

→ Don't overschedule your child

→ Encourage open communication - especially when a big change is to be expected

→ Encourage family routines (we have dinner together every day, we do family fun night every Friday, etc)

- Role model relaxation exercises

M&M MOMENT

Deep Breathing

Mindful deep breathing is one of the best things you and your children can do anytime - when you feel you're getting upset, when you're sad, or when you get hurt. Deep breathing calms your nerves, allows more air into your lungs to circulate more oxygen, and relaxes your muscles.

Close your eyes. Place your hands on your belly. Take a deep breath, inhale through the nose for 3 seconds as you feel your belly expand... Hold for 2 seconds. Blow out for 5 seconds, visualizing all the toxins and stress released from your body. Then say any affirmation - I am strong, I am capable.

For kids: Close your eyes. Inhale to smell the flowers for 3 seconds, blow the candles out for 5 seconds. Then say any affirmation - I can do it, I am strong.

Mantras

Challenge: *Google your favorite mantras and say these OUT LOUD every day upon waking*

I can't change my past. Acknowledge it, forgive myself, and stop worrying about it. Do what I can today, because I **can still change my future!**	Focus on SOLUTIONS, not problems to regain control of the situation	I am loved. I am enough. I have strength. I am fearless. I am strong. I am beautiful. I have faith. I believe in myself.

KID'S TIME TO SHINE

Create an affirmation/vision board for your children. Print out your favorite mantras, put it in their bedrooms, or even write it out on a post-it, and stick it on the bathroom mirrors - wherever they can see it often! Have them repeat these mantras every day. Also, post pictures of what they want to achieve and things that make them happy. Have them meditate on this before bedtime to relieve the small or big daily stressors of life!

☆ Say NO to anything "extra" this week. These days are often overscheduled & sometimes you just need a break. Spend a day discussing your family's values. Ask your children, what do they wish their days looked like?

☐ ☐ ☐ ☐ ☐ ☐ ☐

IN TODAY'S RUSH, WE ALL THINK TOO MUCH, SEEK TOO MUCH, WANT TOO MUCH, AND FORGET ABOUT THE JOY OF JUST BEING

– ECKHART TOLLE

THIS WEEK'S TOP THREE

☆ _____

☆ _____

☆ _____

Sunday

Sleep ☺ 😐 😴

Move your body

Monday

Sleep ☺ 😐 😴

Move your body

Tuesday

Sleep ☺ 😐 😴

Move your body

Wednesday

Sleep ☺ 😐 😫

Move your body

Thursday

Sleep ☺ 😐 😫

Move your body

Friday

Sleep ☺ 😐 😫

Move your body

Saturday

Sleep ☺ 😐 😫

Move your body

A favorite memory that always makes me smile...

☆ Review Nurse's Notes: Happy hormones

☆ Learn and implement ways to increase your happy hormones naturally

☐ ☐ ☐ ☐ ☐ ☐ ☐

THE MIND IS EVERYTHING. WHAT YOU THINK, YOU BECOME

– BUDDHA

THIS WEEK'S TOP THREE

☆ _____

☆ _____

☆ _____

⬡ **Sunday**

Sleep 😊 😐 😴

Move your body

⬡ **Monday**

Sleep 😊 😐 😴

Move your body

⬡ **Tuesday**

Sleep 😊 😐 😴

Move your body

Wednesday

Sleep 🙂 😐 😴

Move your body

Thursday

Sleep 🙂 😐 😴

Move your body

Friday

Sleep 🙂 😐 😴

Move your body

Saturday

Sleep 🙂 😐 😴

Move your body

I am thankful for...

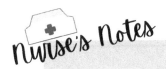

HAPPY HORMONES

These are the hormones that are responsible for making you happy. The more you produce these hormones, the more you are willing to take on the day, decrease stress and improve sleep.

✓ **Dopamine:** aka "happy hormones." This hormone is released by the brain when you experience something pleasurable or when you give or receive a reward.

✓ **Serotonin:** aka "feel-good hormones." This hormone is produced mostly by the gut. it is responsible for stabilizing mood, decreasing the risk of anxiety and depression, and helping with sleep. It can even affect digestion.

✓ **Endorphins:** aka "the runner's high." The hormone most commonly associated with exercise. Aerobics or any exercise that increases heart rate and breathing increases this hormone. They also function as natural pain killers, reduce your perception of pain, increase your ability to cope with illness, and helps with sleep..

✓ **Oxytocin:** aka "the love hormone." This hormone plays a role in bonding and attachment. A woman's body is flooded with this hormone when having a baby and nursing.

> You have control over your emotions. Your thoughts and feelings may come and go like waves in the ocean. But you can absolutely pick out which positive thoughts to hold onto, and which negative ones you want to pass.

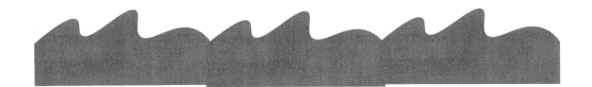

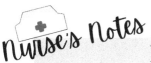
HAPPY HORMONES CONTINUED...

These are natural ways to increase your body's production of happy hormones

─────────────── *Nutrition* ───────────────

→ Adequate protein intake combined with complex carbohydrates are needed to produce the hormones dopamine and serotonin

→ Increase intake of omega 3's, healthy fats, and reduce saturated fats to help balance hormones. Review week 19.

→ Eggs, pineapple, turkey, and nuts have nutrients that produce serotonin

→ Dark chocolate and red wine helps produce endorphins

→ Probiotics, such as yogurt and fermented foods, are needed to improve gut health, which helps produce serotonin

→ Getting adequate vitamin D helps produce serotonin and oxytocin. This can be fulfilled by eating fatty fish, mushrooms, eggs, and being outside for 15 minutes of sunshine!

─────────────── *Lifestyle* ───────────────

- Help someone out
- Daily gratitude
- Receiving praise
- Engaging in your favorite hobby
- Exercise or play
- Spending time outside
- Exposure to sun at least 15 minutes
- Adequate sleep

- Acupuncture/Massage
- Meditation
- Laugh
- Taking a bath
- Cuddling with family or pets
- Listening to music
- Sharing feelings
-Enjoying time with family and friends

MAKE A PLAN Pick 2 things under each category - nutrition and lifestyle - to implement in your family's routine. Which do you choose and how will you implement it? Be specific!

Promise to myself:_____

_____

_____

MONTHLY REFLECTION

Use this time to review your vision board and update as needed!

☆ A moment I can't forget...

☆ The hardest thing about this past month was...

☆ We got through the hardest times together by...

☆ I am so proud of...

☆ Best meal I thouroughly enjoyed:

☆ The funniest thing that happened was...

KID'S TIME TO SHINE

Space for your kids to write or draw what they enjoyed the most this last month

MONTHLY HABIT TRACKER

Print one out for each family member & post it on your family board! Track the habits you are concentrating on. Color it in after completing it and celebrate every day's win! 1 symbol = 1 day.

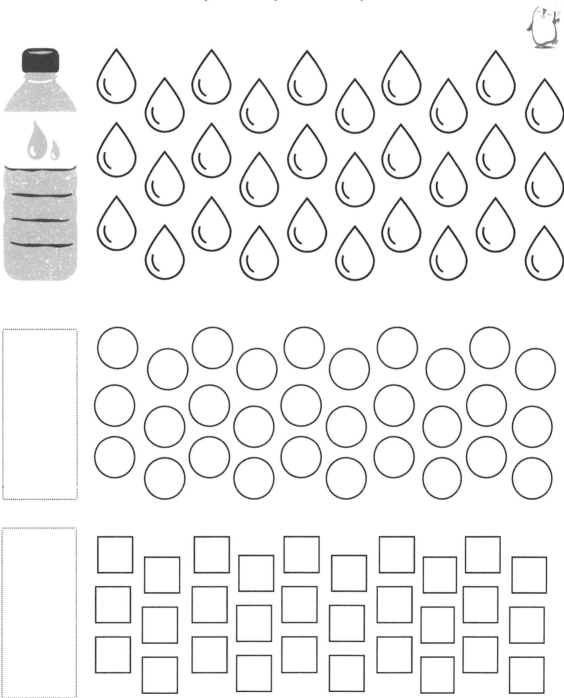

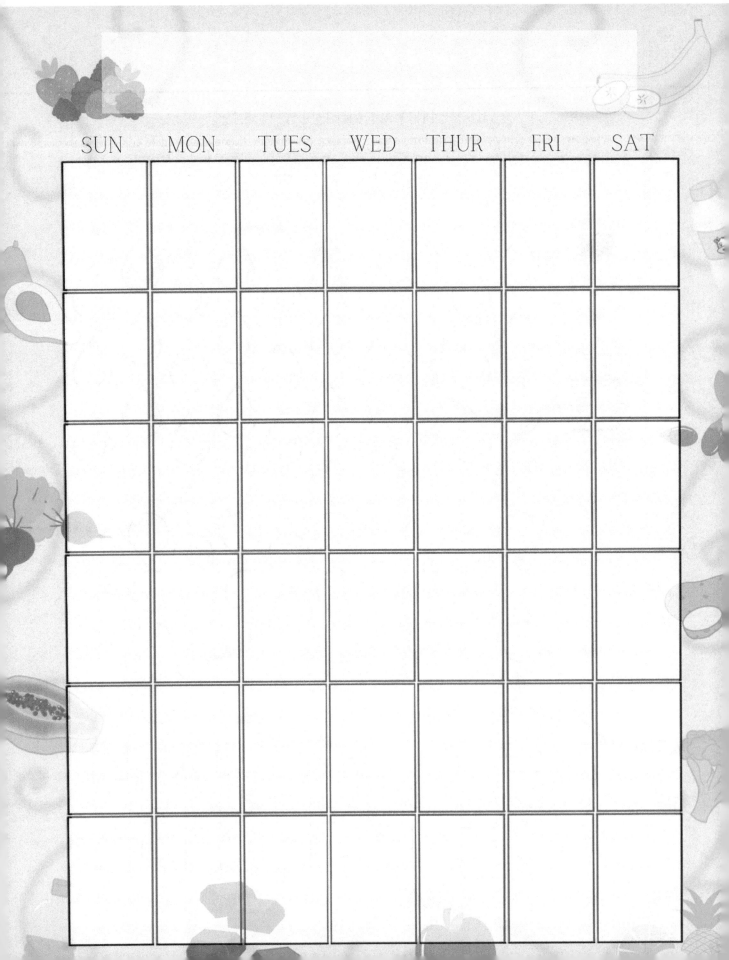

SUN	MON	TUES	WED	THUR	FRI	SAT

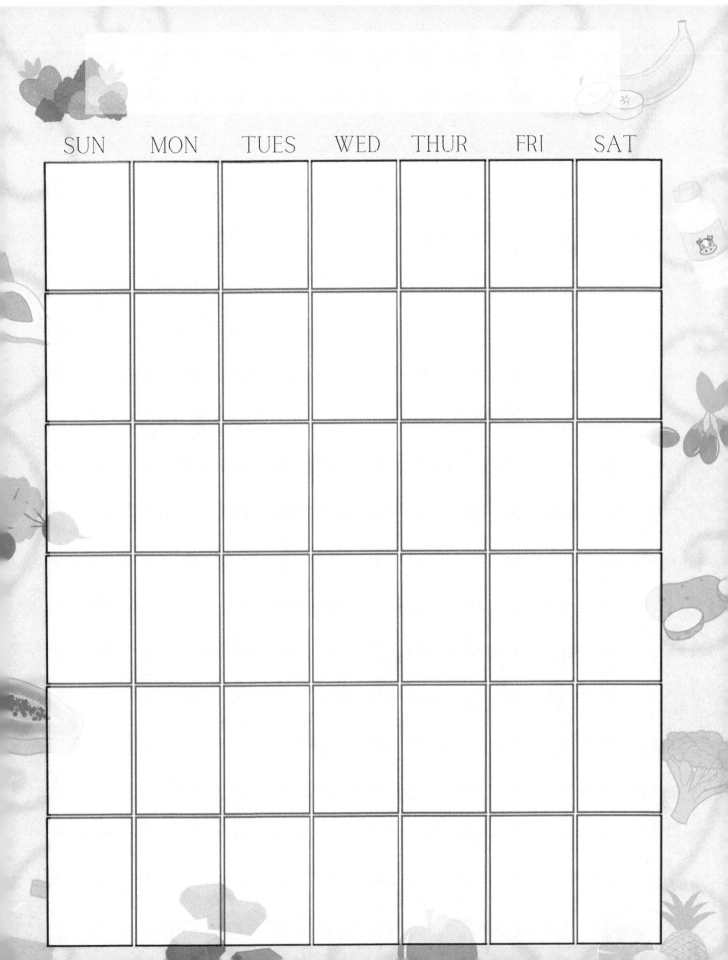

SUN	MON	TUES	WED	THUR	FRI	SAT

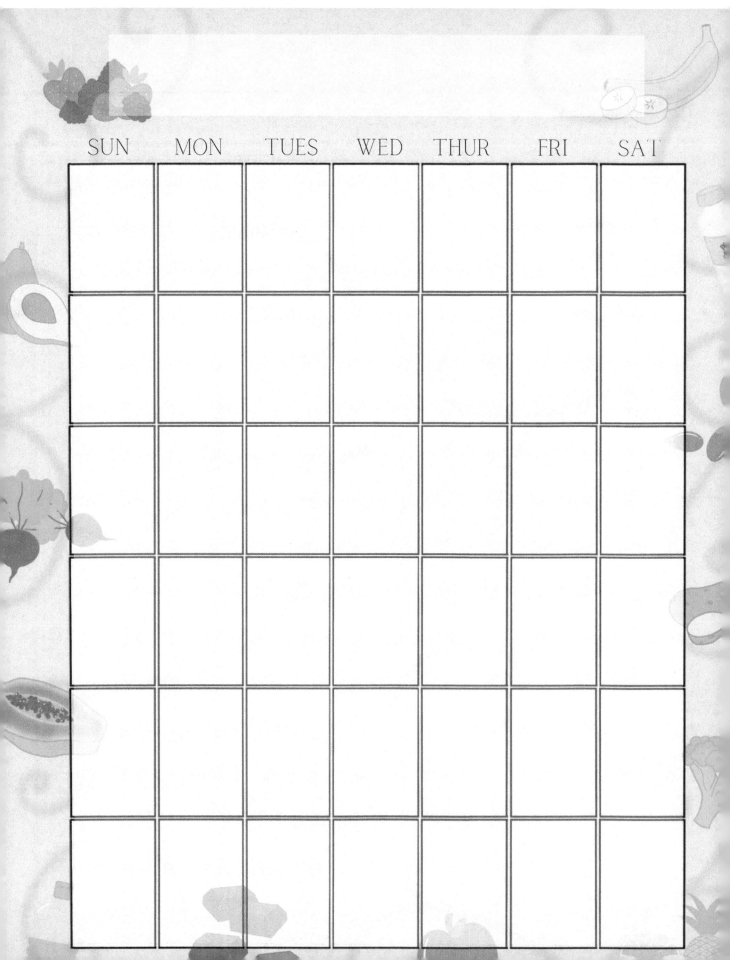

SUN	MON	TUES	WED	THUR	FRI	SAT

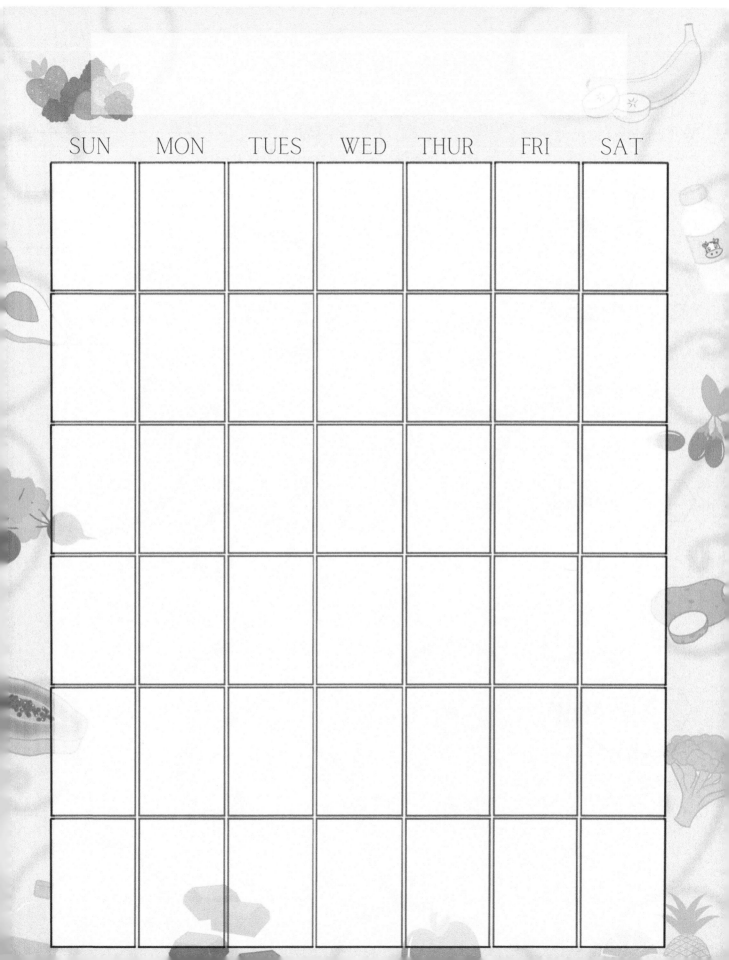

SUN	MON	TUES	WED	THUR	FRI	SAT

WEEK 37 CHALLENGE

☆ Review nurse's notes

☆ Kid's time to shine activity

THE MIND IS LIKE A
MUSCLE – THE MORE
YOU EXERCISE IT, THE
STRONGER IT GETS
AND THE MORE IT CAN
EXPAND

– IDOWU KOYENIKAN

THIS WEEK'S TOP THREE

☆ _____

☆ _____

☆ _____

Sunday

Sleep 🙂 😐 😫

Move your body

Monday

Sleep 🙂 😐 😫

Move your body

Tuesday

Sleep 🙂 😐 😫

Move your body

Wednesday

Sleep 🙂 😐 😴

Move your body

Thursday

Sleep 🙂 😐 😴

Move your body

Friday

Sleep 🙂 😐 😴

Move your body

Saturday

Sleep 🙂 😐 😴

Move your body

Something I handled well...

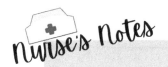

EXERCISE YOUR BRAIN

— Why is brain health important? —

People often exercise their bodies to stay fit, but forget to exercise their brains for healthy aging. Your child's brain grows rapidly in the first five years. Brain development during this time can have a long-term impact on their future health. But it is never too late to start nourishing your brain. Your lifestyle habits and what you eat can continue to improve and maintain the health of your brain significantly.

— Benefits of a healthy brain —

You're happy!

- Improves coordination and balance to prevent falls or injuries
- Healthy brain = strong, resilient brain = able to manage stress and anxiety better
- Decrease risk of anxiety and depression
- Improves concentration, creativity, problem-solving, and productivity

- Protect against memory loss
- Decrease risk of dementia and Alzheimer's Disease
- Decrease risk of headaches and sleep problems
- Able to perform its functions throughout the body more efficiently

— Lifestyle —

→ **Eat healthy carbohydrates and proteins** to fuel the brain. This combination keeps blood sugar stabilized to supply steady energy for the brain. If the blood sugar goes down too fast, brain function decreases as well. Review week 11

→ **Eat to reduce inflammation** and build brain cells to prevent diseases that affect the brain. Review Omega 3's in week 19 and antioxidants in week 21

→ **Stay active**! Exercise increases blood flow to the brain, which improves mood, learning, memory, and lowers the risk of Alzheimer's Disease

→ **Sleep**. Sleeping is when your brain heals itself. It cleans up all the toxins and turns information into long-term memory

→ **Challenge your mind**. Learning new things constantly works out different parts of your brain to create new brain cells and connections

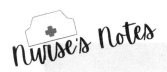

EXERCISE YOUR BRAIN

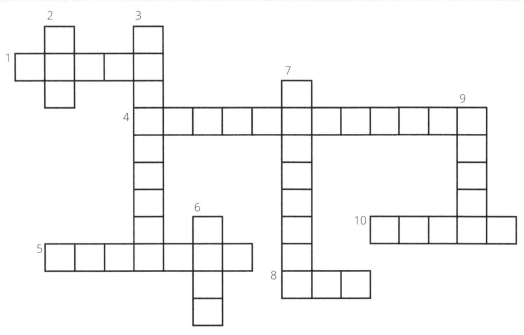

Across

1. Your brain is made up of 70-75% of this liquid. Without it, you can't think clearly, and may even get headaches

4. Free radicals naturally occur after eating, but too much can damage brain cells. What is found in fruits and vegetables that can help clean this up?

5. Eating this macronutrient throughout the day is important to stabilize your blood sugar

8. Your brain's health is directly related to your lifestyle habits and what you _____

10. When your brain is healthy, your emotions are better controlled, and you feel _____ !

Down

2. A good oil change is important to build healthy brain cells because your brain is made up of 60% _____ !

3. Eating this every morning gives your brain the fuel and energy to tackle the day

6. Your child's brain grows the most in the first _____ years

7. Doing this physical activity every day can help increase blood flow to the brain

9. This is the time the brain sorts through memories and heals itself

1. Water. 2. Fat 3. Breakfast. 4. Antioxidants. 5. Protein. 6. Five. 7. Exercise. 8. Eat. 9. Sleep. 10. Happy

KIDS TIME TO SHINE

Find new activities to play that will challenge your family's brain. Learning anything new builds new brain cells and connections! Cooking new recipes, playing card games, jigsaw puzzles, dancing, and using all your senses to describe your environment.

☆ Pick one new habit from previous weeks you still need work on

☐ ☐ ☐ ☐ ☐ ☐ ☐

☆ Send a message to someone each day to express your gratitude.

☐ ☐ ☐ ☐ ☐ ☐ ☐

PRACTICING GRATITUDE ALLOWS YOU TO BUILD A HABIT OF SEEKING AND FINDING THE GOOD IN YOUR LIFE

THIS WEEK'S TOP THREE

☆ _____

☆ _____

☆ _____

Sunday

Sleep 🙂 😐 😴

Move your body

Monday

Sleep 🙂 😐 😴

Move your body

Tuesday

Sleep 🙂 😐 😴

Move your body

Wednesday

Sleep 🙂 😐 😴

Move your body

Thursday

Sleep 🙂 😐 😴

Move your body

Friday

Sleep 🙂 😐 😴

Move your body

Saturday

Sleep 🙂 😐 😴

Move your body

A person I appreciated...

Motivation
IS WHAT GETS
YOU STARTED
Habit
IS WHAT KEEPS
YOU GOING

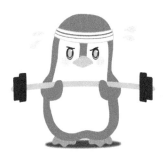

PHASE FOUR

MOVE YOUR BODY

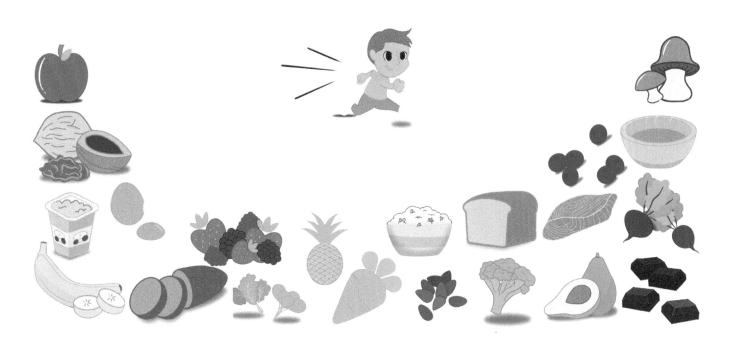

WEEK 39 CHALLENGE

☆ Kids Time to Shine Activity

☆ Review - Power of Play

☆ Are you still eating 3 servings
of vegetables daily?

☐ ☐ ☐ ☐ ☐ ☐ ☐

EXERCISE IS A
CELEBRATION OF WHAT
YOUR BODY CAN DO,
NOT A PUNISHMENT
FOR WHAT YOU ATE.

- WOMEN'S HEALTH UK

THIS WEEK'S TOP THREE

☆ _____

☆ _____

☆ _____

Sunday

Sleep 😊 😐 😣

Move your body

Monday

Sleep 😊 😐 😣

Move your body

Tuesday

Sleep 😊 😐 😣

Move your body

Wednesday

Sleep ☺ 😐 😴

Move your body

Thursday

Sleep ☺ 😐 😴

Move your body

Friday

Sleep ☺ 😐 😴

Move your body

Saturday

Sleep ☺ 😐 😴

Move your body

Something new I learned...

THE POWER OF PLAY

Play is a great way to relieve stress and engage in movement and creativity for adults and children. It is also an opportunity for families to bond, improve communication, and a time for parents to role model that health and family are a priority. More benefits include...

- Play builds strong bones and muscles
- Play promotes a healthy heart
- Play improves metabolism
- Play boosts mood and happy hormones

- Play improves concentration
- Play prevents you from getting sick
- Play improves coordination
- Play improves sleep

Activity Box

- Grab any container (jar or box)
- Make a copy and cut up the pieces on the next page
- Take turns to pick out 1 or 2 surprise activities to choose from
- Do this for at least 30 minutes with a goal of at least 3 times a week!

Bonus tips

→ Don't call it "exercise." Exercise doesn't sound nearly as fun as "let's go play outside!"

→ Get the whole family pedometers so everyone can compete with each other on how many steps they can take in a day.

→ Offer prizes (winner picks the movie on movie night, or the winner gets to choose their favorite dessert/dinner on Saturdays, etc)

→ Even if you have no children, you can find ways to make these activities work! :)

→ Yoga: The best ones to do with children are inversion exercises - child's pose, downward-facing dog, headstands, etc. These in particular are known to activate the "rest and digest" response and restore balance to your nervous system.

→ YouTube is a great resource to fulfill lots of these activities

→ Don't forget to add more of your favorite options!

Freeze dance party	Balloon tennis
Basketball/football	Park/playground
Walk outside/play I spy	Karaoke
Karate on Youtube	Workout on YouTube
Ride bikes	Guided meditation
Hide and seek	Jump rope
Yoga – Inversion	Board games
Painting	Hula hoop
Push up/Sit ups	Animal race
Jumping jacks	Follow the leader
Hopscotch	Pillow fight

☆ Play your favorite upbeat song to wake your family up in the morning. Get up and dance for one song before getting ready or during breakfast time!

☐ ☐ ☐ ☐ ☐ ☐ ☐

WHEN LIFE GETS BLURRY, ADJUST YOUR FOCUS

THIS WEEK'S TOP THREE

☆ _____

☆ _____

☆ _____

Sunday

Sleep 😊 😐 😫

Move your body

Monday

Sleep 😊 😐 😫

Move your body

Tuesday

Sleep 😊 😐 😫

Move your body

Wednesday

Sleep 🙂 😐 😴

Move your body

Thursday

Sleep 🙂 😐 😴

Move your body

Friday

Sleep 🙂 😐 😴

Move your body

Saturday

Sleep 🙂 😐 😴

Move your body

I am proud of myself for...

MONTHLY REFLECTION

Use this time to review your vision board and update as needed!

☆ What were your family's biggest accomplishments?

☆ What were your biggest fears/stressors?

☆ How did you or do you plan on overcoming those fears/stressors?

☆ Have you noticed any changes in your family, such as behavior, symptoms or etc.?

☆ I am so proud of...

☆ The funniest thing that happened was...

KID'S TIME TO SHINE

Space for your kids to write or draw what they enjoyed the most this last month

MONTHLY HABIT TRACKER

Print one out for each family member & post it on your family board! Track the habits you are concentrating on. Color it in after completing it and celebrate every day's win! 1 symbol = 1 day.

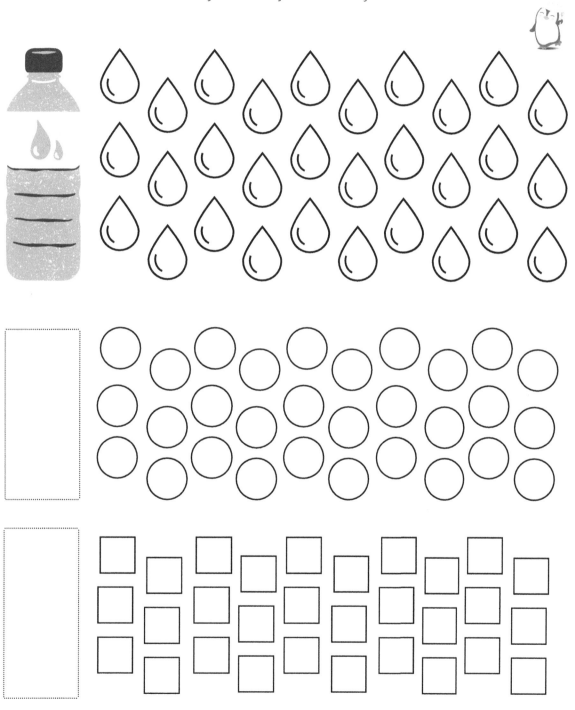

WEEK 41 CHALLENGE

☆ Do 5 isometric exercises at least twice day

☐ ☐ ☐ ☐ ☐ ☐ ☐

☆ Review Nurse's Notes

☆ Make a plan

Motivation
is what gets you started
Habit
is what keeps you going

- Jim Rohn

THIS WEEK'S TOP THREE

☆ _____

☆ _____

☆ _____

Sunday

Sleep 😊 😐 😴

Move your body

Monday

Sleep 😊 😐 😴

Move your body

Tuesday

Sleep 😊 😐 😴

Move your body

Wednesday

Sleep 🙂 😐 😫

Move your body

Thursday

Sleep 🙂 😐 😫

Move your body

Friday

Sleep 🙂 😐 😫

Move your body

Saturday

Sleep 🙂 😐 😫

Move your body

Something that brought me joy...

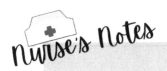

TIME TO MOVE

The best exercise for you is the one you will do - Dr. Sears

There are many different ways you can keep your body moving and prevent muscle loss. No gym or hours on a treadmill is needed! Moving your body helps heal your body and a lot can be done anytime and anywhere. Movement is good for your body as much as it is for your mind! When you learn new moves, it also builds new pathways in your brain to keep it sharp.

—————— Strength Training ——————

The more muscles you have, the more efficient and faster your metabolism will be. You will burn calories even when you're not exercising! Some of the easiest ways to include strength training in your everyday routine are learning **isometric exercises** and having **resistance bands** on hand. These small movements throughout the day can help you stay fit.

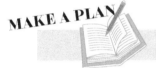

PROMISE TO MYSELF

Google search for more isometric and resistance bands exercises! Where in your daily routine can you sneak them in?

Exercise	Sneak it in!
Heel raises	At least 3 times a day while cooking or preparing food
_____	_____
_____	_____
_____	_____
_____	_____
_____	_____

Isometric exercises

Challenge: *Do 5 isometric exercises at least twice a day*

Isometric exercises are a great way to engage your muscles without using any equipment. This can be done anywhere while sitting at a desk at work or in a classroom without disturbing anyone!

Sample exercises...

- Press your palms together in front of your chest like you're praying, and keep your elbows up so your arms are parallel to the ground. Firmly press them together engaging your arm muscles. Hold this position for 10 seconds, then relax. Repeat 5 times.

- With your elbows still out and your arms parallel to the ground, face one hand palm up, the other palm down, hook together to make an interlocking fist. Pull outwards for 10 seconds, then relax. Repeat 5 times. Switch hands and repeat.

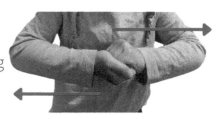

- Suck your belly in to engage your abdominal muscles, tense your glutes and pelvis, like you need to go to the bathroom. Do this 10 seconds at a time. Repeat 5 times.

- When sitting in a chair, cross your lower legs, ankle over the other ankle. Lift legs off the floor and press your upper leg and lower leg against each other - lower leg up and upper leg down, 10 seconds at a time. Repeat 5 times. Switch legs and do this again.

- When you're standing in line at the supermarket, or on the phone, do heel raises 10 seconds at a time. Repeat 5 times.

☆ After eating your biggest meal, walk or play for 10 minutes

☐ ☐ ☐ ☐ ☐ ☐ ☐

☆ Sneak more movement into your day

☐ ☐ ☐ ☐ ☐ ☐ ☐

☆ Kid's time to shine actitvity

Exercise doesn't just change your body, it changes your *mind, attitude, and your mood*

THIS WEEK'S TOP THREE

☆ _____

☆ _____

☆ _____

Sunday

Sleep ☺ 😐 😴

Move your body

Monday

Sleep ☺ 😐 😴

Move your body

Tuesday

Sleep ☺ 😐 😴

Move your body

Wednesday

Sleep ☺ 😐 😩

Move your body

Thursday

Sleep ☺ 😐 😩

Move your body

Friday

Sleep ☺ 😐 😩

Move your body

Saturday

Sleep ☺ 😐 😩

Move your body

A favorite memory that always make me smile...

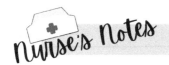

SAY YES TO "NO"

Nitric Oxide

In 1998, Dr. Ignarro won a Nobel Prize for his discovery in the role of Nitric Oxide (NO) gas in our bodies. It helps turn on your body's own internal pharmacy to protect your heart, brain, and more! The best and most consistent way to activate this gas is through exercise. When your breathing and heart rate increase with exercise, nitric oxide is released and further improves the blood flow of oxygen and nutrients to your muscles, organs, and your brain.

✓ Increases antioxidant activity to keep your blood vessels healthy overall
✓ Lowers your blood pressure
✓ Lowers your cholesterol and prevents blood clots
✓ Reduces risk of stroke and heart attack
✓ Increases levels of natural anti-inflammatory to help heal
✓ Improves mood
✓ Strengthens your immune system

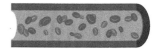

Walking, walking

 Morning: A 10-minute brisk walk outside before breakfast can get you ready for the day. Hormones are released to wake you up, increase energy, burn fat, and improve mood

- Afternoon: A 10-minute brisk walk after your biggest meal of the day can prevent your blood sugar from spiking too high. It can also improve blood flow to the brain so you're sharper and less stressed for the rest of your work/school day

Evening: A brisk walk can relieve the stresses from work/school, help you unwind for your evening routine, and regulate the amount of food you eat for dinner.

*Choose speed over distance - walking faster is more efficient than walking longer

KID'S TIME TO SHINE

One of my toddler's favorite song is "Walking, walking" by Super Simple Songs. This song encourages movement, and is a great song to wake up to! Find your favorite songs to wake up to in the morning

TIME TO MOVE

Challenge: *Sneak more movement into your daily routine*

If you've heard this a lot before, but were hesitant to do it... NOW IS THE TIME! Here are some tips to sneak some extra movement into your day.

✓ Take the stairs instead of the elevator

Start small: If you're on the 5th floor, go up one flight of stairs, and take the elevator for the remaining 4 floors. Then increase the number of stairs as you build up endurance

✓ Park far from entrances

Stop driving back and forth in a parking lot looking for the closest parking! Find the first parking spot you see and just go for it. You save so much more time!

✓ Exercise while watching TV or doing computer work

During commercials, get up! Do 10 jumping jacks and drink some water. If you're on the computer or watching a movie, have exercise bands or small weights in hand. Do 10 reps at least every hour

✓ Do you have stairs in your home? Stairs are a great exercise tool we take for granted in our homes! Use the farthest bathroom in the house, especially if it's up the stairs to get those extra steps in

✓ Doing household chores can be quite an exercise. Make a game out of it with your family - who can clean the bathroom or their rooms the fastest

✓ Wash the car by hand, instead of going to the car wash. It's also much more fun to do with the kids

MAKE A PLAN

What other activities can you and your family do to sneak more movement and steps into your lifestyle?

Promise to myself: _____

_____

WEEK 43 CHALLENGE

☆ Grab your favorite face cream and Youtube "Face exercises." Find your favorite one and do it every morning or evening as part of your routine. We tend to hold a lot of stress in our faces, this will help!

☐ ☐ ☐ ☐ ☐ ☐ ☐

You can do
Anything,
but not everything

THIS WEEK'S TOP THREE

☆ _____

☆ _____

☆ _____

Sunday

Sleep 🙂 😐 😔

Move your body

Monday

Sleep 🙂 😐 😔

Move your body

Tuesday

Sleep 🙂 😐 😔

Move your body

Wednesday

Sleep 🙂 😐 😴

Move your body

Thursday

Sleep 🙂 😐 😴

Move your body

Friday

Sleep 🙂 😐 😴

Move your body

Saturday

Sleep 🙂 😐 😴

Move your body

I am thankful for...

☆ Do these stretches upon waking and before bedtime
☐ ☐ ☐ ☐ ☐ ☐ ☐

☆ Are you still drinking enough water?
☐ ☐ ☐ ☐ ☐ ☐ ☐

☆ Kid's time to shine activity

Your body is a reflection of your
Lifestyle

THIS WEEK'S TOP THREE

☆ _____

☆ _____

☆ _____

Sunday

Sleep ☺ 😐 😴

Move your body

Monday

Sleep ☺ 😐 😴

Move your body

Tuesday

Sleep ☺ 😐 😴

Move your body

Wednesday

Sleep 🙂 😐 😴

Move your body

Thursday

Sleep 🙂 😐 😴

Move your body

Friday

Sleep 🙂 😐 😴

Move your body

Saturday

Sleep 🙂 😐 😴

Move your body

Something I handled well...

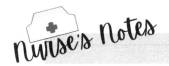

TIME TO MOVE

─── Flexibility ───

Flexibility exercises include stretches, yoga, and some pilates. These loosen and lengthen your muscles, which can lower your risk of developing arthritis and joint problems as you age. Incorporating simple yoga poses into your morning routine can increase your focus and energy throughout the day. Simple yoga poses that are done in the evening can help activate your calming hormones for a better night's sleep.

─── Yoga ───

 Morning upon waking

- While lying on your bed, bring your arms above your head, hold your left wrist with your right hand and gently pull to stretch your arms. Stretch 10 seconds at a time. Switch arms. Repeat at least 2 times on each side.

- Roll onto your stomach and into a **child's pose**. Hold for 10 seconds.

- Slowly get up and move onto the floor for more stability. Position yourself into a **downward-facing dog**. Hold for 10 seconds.

- Either on the floor or sitting up on the bed, twist your body to stretch your sides. Hold for 10 seconds. Repeat at least 2 times on each side.

 Evening before going to bed

- While lying in bed or on the floor, sit upright, bring your knees up together to hug. With your feet together, let your knees open to the sides creating the **butterfly pose**. Close your eyes and focus on your breathing. Do breathing exercises from Week 32, at least 3 times.

- Lay on your back and bring your legs up against the wall. Close your eyes and do breathing exercises at least 3 times. Relax for total of 3-5 minutes or as long as you can tolerate.

LAUGHTER IS THE BEST MEDICINE

When was the last time you laughed so hard, you had tears running down your face? Laughing gives every part of your body a good workout. Surround yourself around positive people who make you laugh.

Brain: Releases happy hormones and can reduce feelings of depression and anxiety. Stress hormones also decrease, and can even temporarily relieve pain

Immune system: White blood cells, the ones responsible for fighting diseases, and cancer-fighting cells increase during laughter

Heart: Laughter increases heart rate and blood flow like you just did an aerobic workout

Lungs: Laughter gives the lung's muscles, the diaphragm, a good workout

Muscles: Relaxes the whole body by relieving muscle tension

KID'S TIME TO SHINE

Spend some time to discuss this with your family. You will be surprised at the awesome ideas your kids come up with. Kids tend to say and do the funniest things!

What movie(s) or show(s) ALWAYS make you laugh? Assign one day a week or month to watch this!

_____

_____

Recall a memory that ALWAYS make you laugh.

_____

_____

_____

MONTHLY REFLECTION

Use this time to review your vision board and update as needed!

☆ A moment I can't forget...

☆ The hardest thing about this past month was...

☆ We got through the hardest times together by...

☆ I am so proud of...

☆ Best meal I thouroughly enjoyed:

☆ The funniest thing that happened was...

KID'S TIME TO SHINE

Space for your kids to write or draw what they enjoyed the most this last month

MONTHLY HABIT TRACKER

Print one out for each family member & post it on your family board! Track the habits you are concentrating on. Color it in after completing it and celebrate every day's win! 1 symbol = 1 day.

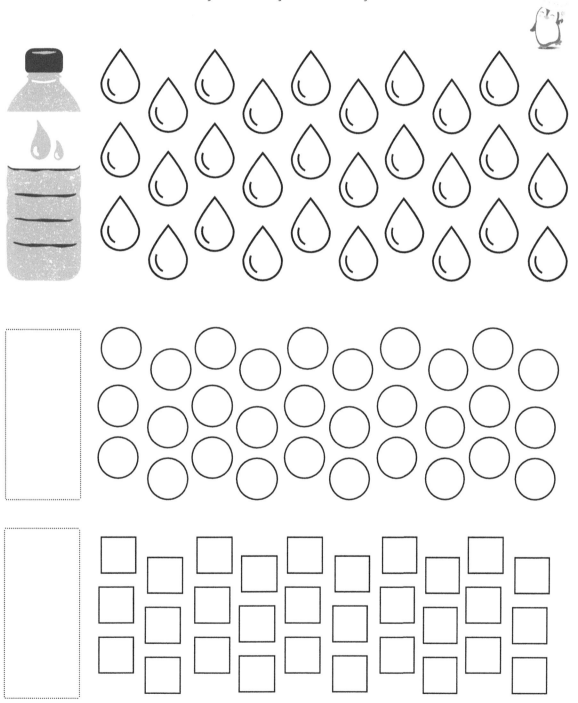

WEEK 45 CHALLENGE

☆ Search YouTube to find your top 3 favorite exercise influencers. My favorite is Blogilates :)

☆ Which were your favorite exercises? Set your intentions and write out a daily routine to follow. Post it on your family board

The only bad workout is *the one you didn't do*

THIS WEEK'S TOP THREE

☆ _____

☆ _____

☆ _____

Sunday

Sleep ☺ 😐 😴

Move your body

Monday

Sleep ☺ 😐 😴

Move your body

Tuesday

Sleep ☺ 😐 😴

Move your body

Wednesday

Sleep 🙂 😐 😫

Move your body

Thursday

Sleep 🙂 😐 😫

Move your body

Friday

Sleep 🙂 😐 😫

Move your body

Saturday

Sleep 🙂 😐 😫

Move your body

A person I appreciated...

WEEK 46 CHALLENGE

☆ Review Nurse's Notes

☆ Repeat these affirmations
to start your day with
positive energy!

☐ ☐ ☐ ☐ ☐ ☐ ☐

IF YOU THINK
WELLNESS
IS EXPENSIVE, TRY
ILLNESS

THIS WEEK'S TOP THREE

☆ _____

☆ _____

☆ _____

⬡ *Sunday*

Sleep 🙂 😐 😫

Move your body

⬡ *Monday*

Sleep 🙂 😐 😫

Move your body

⬡ *Tuesday*

Sleep 🙂 😐 😫

Move your body

Wednesday

Sleep 🙂 😐 😴

Move your body

Thursday

Sleep 🙂 😐 😴

Move your body

Friday

Sleep 🙂 😐 😴

Move your body

Saturday

Sleep 🙂 😐 😴

Move your body

Something new I learned...

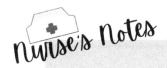

ENERGY BOOST

Challenge: *Reflect on these notes and assess where your family can make changes*

Clean eating, and removing the harmful chemicals in your diet is an important step to take when improving your energy levels. Hopefully, by now, you have noticed better energy levels in your family from before you started this planner! But if you still often find yourself feeling fatigued or tired, or your children wake up irritable and not ready to take on the day, here are some key nutrients to consider and lifestyle habits to reassess...

✓ **Nutrition:** Any food you eat provides calories, which provides energy. But not all foods are created equal in how long that energy lasts. Focus on eating complex carbohydrates with fiber, proteins, and fats for long-lasting energy and stable blood sugar. This combination keeps your brain alert. Simple carbohydrates increase energy fast but leave you feeling sluggish shortly after. Review week 11 and week 13.

✓ **Key nutrients for an energy boost**

- Iron: Helps bring oxygen to all parts of your body to give it energy. Found in lentils, spinach, fortified whole-grain cereals, turkey, chicken, quinoa, and more

- B vitamins: A deficiency in some of the B vitamins can lead to fatigue, and decreased mood. B vitamins are found in lean meats, nuts and seeds

- Prebiotics/Probiotics: Food for your gut. If your gut is not well-fed, it can cause inflammation. This inflammation can prevent the proper absorption of nutrients. So, you may be eating the right foods for energy, but your body can't use it! Review week 22

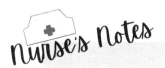

ENERGY BOOST CONTINUED.

✓ **Hydration:** Remember, your bodies are mostly made up of water. If you're not hydrating enough during the day, your brain and body cannot function effectively, and you'll feel sluggish. Review week 4.

✓ **Sleep**: Are you getting enough sleep at nighttime?

- Adults and teenagers need at least 7 hours of sleep, school-aged children need 10+ hours, toddlers and infants 11+ hours

✓ **Exercise:** Even though you may be too tired to get in those daily steps, lack of exercise could be contributing to fatigue. Movement and play give a boost in your body's hormones that help improve mental health, daytime fatigue, and your sleep at night

✓ **Mental health:** If you're not getting enough nutrients, hydration, sleep, or exercise, this can lead to imbalanced hormones → which causes stress, low energy levels, and brain fog! Everything is connected to everything. On the other hand, if you have chronic stress, depression, anxiety, or other mental health imbalances, this can absolutely affect your energy levels also. We discuss some simple ways to manage these, but please seek out support from your community and your provider to help! In the meantime, *repeat these affirmations for positive energy each morning.*

I am strong. I am gifted. I am grateful. I am fearless. I am worthy. I am enough. I am blessed.	I am in control of my own energy. I can choose how I feel in every moment.	I am grateful for this beautiful day. I will find goodness in all things. I have the power to rise above negativity that do not serve me. I am capable of great things today.

WEEK 47 CHALLENGE

☆ Get fresh air and sunlight first thing in the morning, at least 5-10 minutes. This helps release the hormones that wake you up and prepare for the day.

☐ ☐ ☐ ☐ ☐ ☐ ☐

☆ Do 30 arm circles outside

IF YOU WANT SOMETHING YOU NEVER HAD, YOU MUST BE WILLING TO DO SOMETHING YOU'VE NEVER DONE

~ THOMAS JEFFERSON

THIS WEEK'S TOP THREE

☆ _____

☆ _____

☆ _____

Sunday

Sleep 😊 😐 😴

Move your body

Monday

Sleep 😊 😐 😴

Move your body

Tuesday

Sleep 😊 😐 😴

Move your body

Wednesday

Sleep 🙂 😐 😴

Move your body

Thursday

Sleep 🙂 😐 😴

Move your body

Friday

Sleep 🙂 😐 😴

Move your body

Saturday

Sleep 🙂 😐 😴

Move your body

I am thankful for...

☆ Pick one new habit from previous weeks you still need work on

☐ ☐ ☐ ☐ ☐ ☐ ☐

☆ Send a message to someone each day to express your gratitude.

☐ ☐ ☐ ☐ ☐ ☐ ☐

DO GOOD.
AND GOOD WILL
COME TO YOU

THIS WEEK'S TOP THREE

☆ _____

☆ _____

☆ _____

Sunday

Sleep ☺ 😐 😕

Move your body

Monday

Sleep ☺ 😐 😕

Move your body

Tuesday

Sleep ☺ 😐 😕

Move your body

Wednesday

Sleep 🙂 😐 😞

Move your body

Thursday

Sleep 🙂 😐 😞

Move your body

Friday

Sleep 🙂 😐 😞

Move your body

Saturday

Sleep 🙂 😐 😞

Move your body

I am proud of myself for...

MONTHLY REFLECTION

Use this time to review your vision board and update as needed!

☆ What were your family's biggest accomplishments?

☆ What were your biggest fears/stressors?

☆ How did you or do you plan on overcoming those fears/stressors?

☆ Have you noticed any changes in your family, such as behavior, symptoms or etc.?

☆ I am so proud of...

☆ Best meal I thouroughly enjoyed:

KID'S TIME TO SHINE

Space for your kids to write or draw what they enjoyed the most this last month

MONTHLY HABIT TRACKER

Print one out for each family member & post it on your family board! Track the habits you are concentrating on. Color it in after completing it and celebrate every day's win! 1 symbol = 1 day.

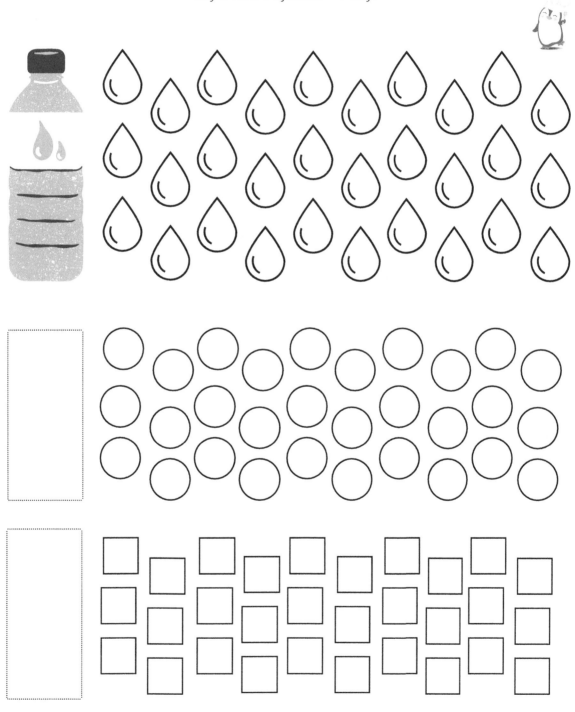

Gratitude

MAKES SENSE OF THE PAST, BRINGS PEACE FOR TODAY, AND CREATES VISION FOR TOMORROW

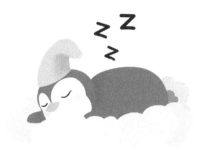

PHASE FIVE

SLEEP

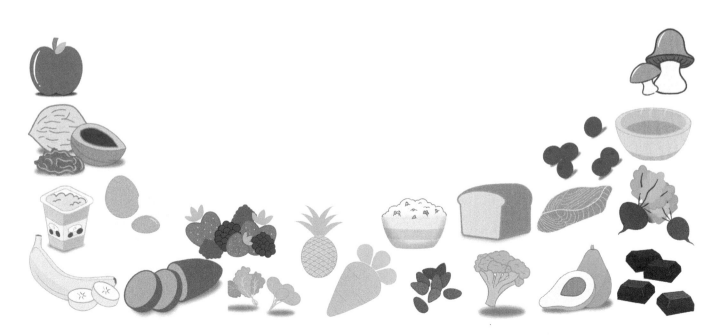

☆ Review nurse's notes: Sleep

☆ Everyone clean your rooms this week! Seriously, tidy it up in a way to create a peaceful environment for sleep

THE SOUL ALWAYS KNOWS WHAT TO DO TO HEAL ITSELF. THE CHALLENGE IS TO SILENCE THE MIND

– CAROLINE MISS

THIS WEEK'S TOP THREE

☆ _____

☆ _____

☆ _____

Sunday

Sleep 🙂 😐 😫

Move your body

Monday

Sleep 🙂 😐 😫

Move your body

Tuesday

Sleep 🙂 😐 😫

Move your body

Wednesday

Sleep 🙂 😐 😴

Move your body

Thursday

Sleep 🙂 😐 😴

Move your body

Friday

Sleep 🙂 😐 😴

Move your body

Saturday

Sleep 🙂 😐 😴

Move your body

Something that brought me joy...

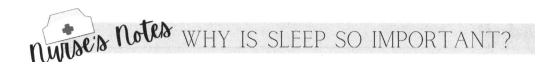

A good night's sleep

Quality sleep is so important to your overall well-being. During sleep...

✓ Turns up the parasympathetic nervous system (review Week 31)

✓ The body repairs worn-out cells

✓ The muscles and organs relax

✓ Heartbeat and breathing slows down

✓ Improves immune system by creating immune cells that fight infection, cancer cells, and inflammation

✓ Regulates emotion and decrease stress hormones

Important for brain health

While the rest of your body is resting, your brain is hard at work...

✓ Organizes new information and the events of the day

✓ Converts memories into long-term memories or erase unneeded information

✓ Removes toxic waste

✓ *When your brain is given time to work efficiently through the night, you will have a clear brain during the day to be focused, make better decisions, improve problem-solving skills and increase creativity!*

Inadequate sleep

Not enough hours of sleep, or restless sleep leads to...

✗ Increases stress hormone and inability to handle stressful events

✗ Increases risk of depression and anxiety

✗ Increases hormones that stimulate appetite, which leads to overeating

✗ Decreases immune system function - increases the risk of inflammation, sickness, and even cancer

✗ Brain fog and fatigue

✗ Inadequate sleep create a vicious cycle - all these reasons above cause hormone imbalance, which causes more sleep difficulties such as restless sleeping and insomnia

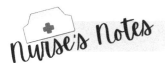

TIME TO REST

Challenge: *Clean your room today! Seriously, let's create a sleep sanctuary for you*

Part of activating your parasympathetic nervous system is using all 5 of our senses to create a peaceful environment to relax in. What's better than visualization? Having your own sleep sanctuary! Your bedroom and/or bathroom should be your own calm-down space. Use your bedroom for sleep only, no work! Here are some ideas to try out.

—— Anatomy of a peaceful sleep environment ——

SIGHT

- Clean and tidied up room
- Candles
- Plants
- Eye mask
- Blackout curtains
- Photos or wall art that sparks joy
- Soft lighting

SMELL

- Lavender and/or Jasmine scented lotions
- Essential oils diffuser
- Essential oil drops/spray on pillow
- Wash pillow cases weekly for freshness

TOUCH

- Cool room temperature, fan or air conditioner near bed
- Warm clothes
- Your favorite bedsheets and blankets that make you feel cozy

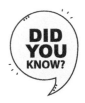

DID YOU KNOW?

Multiple studies have shown that indoor plants are an amazing addition to any room! They improve air quality, and have a psychological and physical impact on your health - making you happier and healthier!

TASTE

- Brush your teeth and floss! Seriously, a super clean mouth will make you feel good through the night

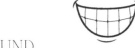

SOUND

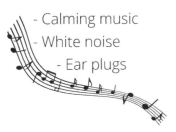

- Calming music
- White noise
- Ear plugs

Set up your bedside table with your necessities, so you don't have to get up often before bed or in the middle of the night...
- Bedside lamp, so you can switch it off from your bed
- Phone, charger
- Book

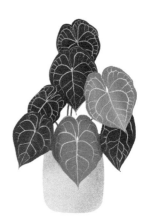

WEEK 50 CHALLENGE

☆ Create a bedtime routine

☐ ☐ ☐ ☐ ☐ ☐

☆ Review week 18. Are you still adding a serving of Omega 3's each day?

☐ ☐ ☐ ☐ ☐ ☐

It never gets easier...
You just get better

THIS WEEK'S TOP THREE

☆ _____

☆ _____

☆ _____

Sunday

Sleep 🙂 😐 😴

Move your body

Monday

Sleep 🙂 😐 😴

Move your body

Tuesday

Sleep 🙂 😐 😴

Move your body

Wednesday

Sleep 🙂 😐 😴

Move your body

Thursday

Sleep 🙂 😐 😴

Move your body

Friday

Sleep 🙂 😐 😴

Move your body

Saturday

Sleep 🙂 😐 😴

Move your body

A favorite memory that always make me smile...

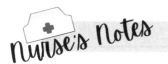

TIME TO REST

Challenge: *Create a bedtime routine*

Humans are creatures of habits. Babies and kids thrive on repetition and routine. A regular schedule provides structure, which supports their emotional development to help them to feel safe and secure. This is helpful for adults too! Creating a structured bedtime routine is similar to telling your body it's almost time to eat (review week 7), your body begins to create the hormones it needs to wind down for peaceful sleep.

— Bedtime Routine Ideas —

HELPS RELEASE SLEEP HORMONES
- Turn off the blue light on phones
- Dim lights in bedrooms
- Complex carbohydrate, small protein, and calcium for dinner
- Chamomile tea, milk

HELPS RELIEVE "THINKING TOO MUCH" THAT DELAYS FALLING ASLEEP
- Journal: a reflection of the day, plan for tomorrow, gratitude moment
- Make a to-do list
- List of unsolved problems (writing this out helps prevent tossing and turning about it through the night, and may help your brain find a solution with good rest!)
- Prepare your clothes and backpack/bag for tomorrow
- Discuss the top 3 things of the day - one good thing, one bad/difficult thing, one random thing

IMPROVE RELAXATION TO WIND DOWN
- No more caffeine after lunchtime
- Have dinner at least 3 hours before bedtime
- Read 5 pages of your favorite book
- Bedtime story with kids
- Guided meditation/deep breathing
- Bedtime stretches/yoga
- Bath, brush/floss teeth
- Music
- Cuddles with kids

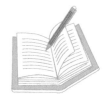

Good sleep depends on what you do during the day. What you do with your body and brain during the day influences how well your body and brain sleep at night.

DAYTIME
- Draw a clear line between day and evening
- No "work" in the bedroom, bedroom only created for rest and sleep
- Open the curtains upon waking to let light in
- Make your bed each morning
- Designate a time bedtime starts
- Get at least 10 minutes of exercise

MY BEDTIME ROUTINE

Use tips from last week and this week to create a bedtime routine for you and your family. In the next several weeks, we will practice optimizing your bedtime routine. Help your kids create a routine for themselves also. Post it in their rooms so they know what to expect.

Did you know?
Getting 15-20 min of sunlight in the morning releases hormones that can dramatically improve your quality of sleep?

Barriers to good sleep

What are your barriers to good sleep? What do you find will be the hardest thing to implement? Write this down, and sleep on it! Identifying and acknowledging it is the first step to healing and finding a solution.

☆ Avoid stressors from your tv/phone at night, at least 30 minutes before bedtime. Stimulation from news and social media, plus blue light exposure overloads the brain and makes it difficult to sleep

☐ ☐ ☐ ☐ ☐ ☐ ☐

Success is a decision

THIS WEEK'S TOP THREE

☆ _____

☆ _____

☆ _____

Sunday

Sleep 🙂 😐 😴

Move your body

Monday

Sleep 🙂 😐 😴

Move your body

Tuesday

Sleep 🙂 😐 😴

Move your body

Wednesday

Sleep 🙂 😐 😴

> Move your body

Thursday

Sleep 🙂 😐 😴

> Move your body

Friday

Sleep 🙂 😐 😴

> Move your body

Saturday

Sleep 🙂 😐 😴

> Move your body

I am thankful for...

WEEK 52 CHALLENGE

☆ Buy comfortable pajamas and/or blankets for everyone that will make you excited to sleep in
☆ Reduce mental stress. When you wake up, spend the first few minutes deep breathing and repeat your daily affirmations

☐ ☐ ☐ ☐ ☐ ☐ ☐

THE STRUGGLE IS PART OF THE JOURNEY

THIS WEEK'S TOP THREE

☆ _____

☆ _____

☆ _____

⬡ **Sunday**

Sleep 🙂 😐 😴

Move your body

⬡ **Monday**

Sleep 🙂 😐 😴

Move your body

⬡ **Tuesday**

Sleep 🙂 😐 😴

Move your body

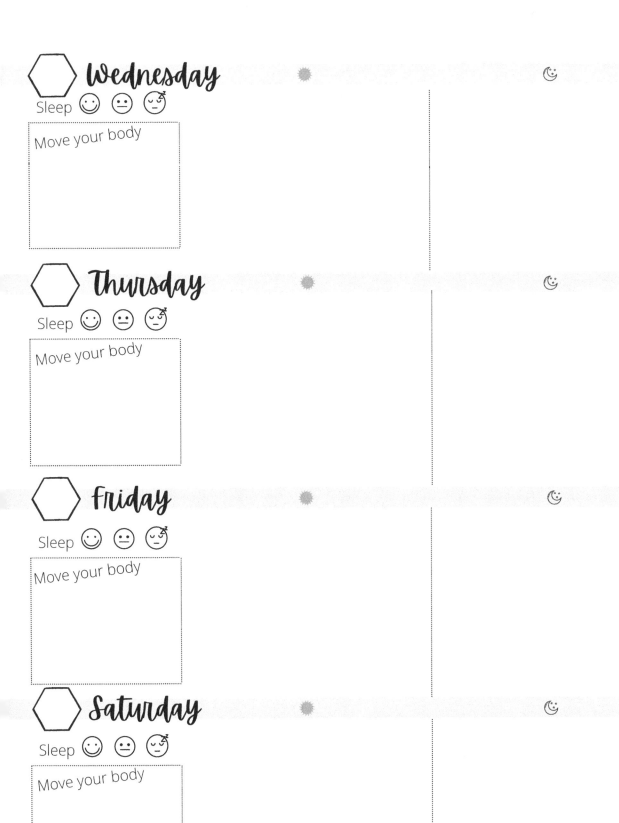

Wednesday

Sleep 🙂 😐 😴

Move your body

Thursday

Sleep 🙂 😐 😴

Move your body

Friday

Sleep 🙂 😐 😴

Move your body

Saturday

Sleep 🙂 😐 😴

Move your body

Something I handled well..

Congratulations

Can you believe it's been ONE YEAR since you started your journey? Look how far you have come! It may not have been perfect and it sure wasn't easy, but I know you and your family have grown exponentially through this whole process. Revisit this journal often to refine and strengthen those healthy habits. Continue to be active in our online community. There is always still something new to learn! Continue to lead by example. I hope that investing in your health becomes a lifelong hobby. Take control of your health and wellness, and it will last for generations!
Good luck on your journey

I GIVE YOU THE GIFT OF HEALTH
- DR. SEARS

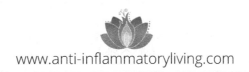

Cover illustrated by Blacy, IG: lacedartanddesign

*Disclaimer: Always seek consultation with your health care provider before starting any new diets or if you have questions regarding your symptoms or medical conditions. The content is not intended to replace medical advice, diagnosis or treatment. The information presented is solely for your education and entertainment purposes.

Made in the USA
Coppell, TX
06 May 2022

77488242R20136